SCULPTING STRENGTH

Unveiling the Power of Nutrition, Bodybuilding, and Steroids

JONATHAN WRIGHT

For permission requests, write to the publisher at the address Premium Book Publishers 15500 Voss Road, Suite 603, Sugar Land, TX 77498

Visit our website: www.premiumbookpublishers.com

First Edition: January 2024

Book Published by Mr. Bracken Joseph on behalf of Premium Book Publishers.

ACKNOWLEDGMENTS

I would like to thank my girlfriend Nadgelli Vazquez for supporting me in
everything that I do.
I would also like to thank all of my Facebook friends and family for
supporting Minotaur Nutrition.

CONTENTS

INTRODUCTION 1

1 Building Blocks of Muscular Marvels 3

2 Shedding Pounds, Gaining Confidence 13

3 Workouts That Work Wonders 23

High-Intensity Interval Training (HIIT) - The Fast Track to Fitness Excellence 27

Fueling Your HIIT Journey 29

Strength Training - Forging a Powerful Physique 30

Cardiovascular/Aerobic Exercise - Unleashing the Power of the Heart and Lungs 33

Yoga - The Harmony of Body and Mind 36

CrossFit - A Holistic Fitness Revolution 39

Maximizing Fitness Gains with Circuit Training 41

Calisthenics: A Dive into Bodyweight Fitness Excellence 46

Martial Arts: Unveiling the Art of Discipline and Strength 50

4 Dive into Diets: From Keto to Kettlebells 57

High-Protein Food Types 62

Keto Diet (Ketogenic Diet) 64

Balanced Macronutrient Diet 66

Intermittent Fasting 67

Plant-Based Diet 69

Paleo Diet 71

Mediterranean Diet 72

Low-Carb Diet 74

5 Steroids: Unveiling the Science 78

Steroids and Their Role in Bodybuilding 81

Understanding How Steroids Interact with Your Biology 84

The Choices, the Consequences, and Finding Your Stance 87

6 Debunking Myths and Embracing Truths 91

7 Amplifying Gains: Legal Supplements for the Win 102

8 The Journey's End and New Beginnings 111

ABOUT THE AUTHOR 117

INTRODUCTION

Hi my name is Jonathan Wright. I decided to write this book for a few reasons. Over the last 25 years I have had a lot of people ask me questions about bodybuilding, nutrition and especially steroids which is the main reason for me writing this. I am not a big guy by any means but I have always found it easy to change my body very quickly. I started out as a personal training through NFPT before I even started to really work on my own body. I'm glad I did though because it gave me much more insight on what would later become a bodybuilder physique. I went from a skinny little bitch to stepping on bodybuilding stages in 2003. I now own my own supplement company called Minotaur Nutrition which I will plug throughout this book lol. Hey can you blame me? Well let's get into what this thing will be about. I'm gonna teach you the real truth about weight loss, supplements, Muscle gaining and yes

STEROIDS! You will learn calorie intake, what to eat and when to eat to achieve your goals. You will learn how to gain muscle as fast as possible. You will learn how to trick your body with simple science to make your goals achievable and yes you will learn about the ins and outs of using anabolic steroids. In no way am I a DR. or nutritionist but I do know alot about these subjects and I'm willing to share this knowledge with you. In no way shape or form is this book telling you what to eat, what to take or what to put into your body. What you do with your body is your own decision. I believe people should know the truth about these subjects because they are very misunderstood. You have been lied to your whole life on how to lose weight. You have been lied to your life on how to gain muscle and you have definitely been lied to about steroids. So come with me on a brief journey into my little world of what we call fitness. If you learn one thing. I have achieved my goal. Thank you for purchasing my book and don't forget to check out minotaurnutrition.com to get the best tasting and baddest ass supplements on the planet!

1 BUILDING BLOCKS OF MUSCULAR MARVELS

All the iron-pumping at the gym isn't doing the job for you. You're worried about not working out hard enough, extra sets, more sweat, and added days in the gym aren't doing the job too; that's not the problem here! The key here is not having the apt knowledge of what to do and what not to do.

Hold on to your seats, folks, because we're about to dive headfirst into the awe-inspiring world of muscles – those unsung champions of our bodies! We're talking about over 600 of these mighty powerhouses, silently making up one-third to one-half of your body weight. Yes, you heard that right; these muscles are no slackers; they're the real muscle-bound MVPs, holding you together, helping you strut your stuff, and ensuring you move through life with style.

Now, even if you're not a card-carrying member of the "Gym Rat" club or a self-proclaimed bodybuilding enthusiast, here's a little secret: your muscles crave attention. Why, you ask? Believe it or not, how you treat these muscular marvels daily can determine whether they wither away or bulk up like they're auditioning for a superhero role. So, picture this: you're standing before a door, ready to unleash your inner action hero. Your brain is like a master conductor, orchestrating the intricate symphony of your muscles. It sends signals to motor neurons in your arm, and they, my friends, are the eager musicians of this orchestra.

On receiving their cue, these neurons set off a spectacular chain reaction, causing your muscles to contract and relax in perfect harmony, leading to the graceful motion that opens the door. But here's the plot twist: the bigger the challenge, the louder the brain's musical score becomes. It calls in more muscle units to join the performance, ensuring you have all the firepower you need to conquer your mission. What if that door felt like it was made of solid iron? Your puny arm muscles might raise the white flag, but your brain isn't giving up that easily.

It rallies other forces to the rescue. You dig in, brace your feet, and summon the power from your core and back muscles to open that door. It's like a battle cry from your body, saying, "I've got this!"

But here's where the plot thickens – while this muscle masterpiece is in full swing, something incredible is happening at the cellular level. Your muscle fibers are experiencing microscopic damage. And you know what? In this context, damage is good, like battle scars that make you more challenging. In response, the injured muscle cells release a posse of inflammatory molecules called cytokines, and these are like the cavalry, swooping in to activate your body's immune system for some serious repair work. This is when the enchanting magic of muscle building unfurls its wings.

The more stress your muscles endure, the more your body gears up for this repair mission. It's like a superhero's secret lair, ready to act. This cycle of damage and repair is the secret sauce behind making your muscles more extensive and more substantial as they adapt to ever-increasing challenges. But here's the kicker: our bodies are already experts at everyday activities. So, if you aim to level up those muscles and become a sculpted marvel, you've got to crank up the resistance – that's the golden ticket to muscle growth. Otherwise, they'll start shrinking in a process known as the muscle atrophy rollercoaster.

But muscles are demanding little divas; they're not

just about action. They're the VIPs who insist on proper nutrition, a hormone-balanced cocktail, and some well-deserved R&R. Think of protein as their building material — it's the Lego set they need to construct those muscle masterpieces. And where do they get it? From the food you eat, of course! Hormones like insulin-like growth factor and testosterone? They're like the personal trainers giving you the pep talk to hit the gym for repair and growth. Oh, and the magic? It happens when you're in dreamland, especially at night. So, if you've ever wondered why sleep is so precious, now you know the answer.

But wait, there's more! The muscle-building game isn't a one-size-fits-all adventure. Gender, age, and even the cards you were dealt genetically can be your secret allies or formidable foes. With their testosterone levels soaring like superhero capes, young men often have a head start in the muscle-building marathon. Genetics also come into play — some lucky individuals have a superhero-like immune response to muscle damage, making them muscle-building champs.

In a nutshell, your body is like that supportive friend who rises to the occasion when you throw challenges its way. Tear up those muscles, feed them right, give them some quality rest, and voila! You've just created the perfect conditions for muscles that aren't just big but also rock-solid strong. It's a bit like life itself – if you want to grow, you've got to embrace challenges and stress because that's where the real magic happens. So, let's unravel the mysteries of muscle growth and embark on this epic journey of discovery together!

***

Now that we are ready for a superb fitness journey, to begin with let's break down the muscle fiber party – we've got red fast twitch, red slow twitch, and the elusive white fibers. Think of them as the three amigos of muscle building, each with unique superpowers.

So, first up, we've got the red slow twitch fibers. These are the marathon runners of the muscle world. They're built for endurance, like those who can run for miles without sweat. To activate these bad boys, you need to engage in activities that require sustained effort over a long period – think long-distance running, cycling, or swimming. They're all about steady, consistent action.

Next in line, we've got the red fast twitch fibers. These are like the sprinters of the muscle world. They're all about explosive bursts of power – think Usain Bolt sprinting down the track or a boxer throwing a knockout punch. To awaken these, you need activities that demand quick, intense bursts of energy, like running, jumping, or lifting heavy weights.

Now, let's talk about the mysterious white fibers,

the muscle ninjas that can do a bit of everything. They're versatile, but they're also a bit lazy. You see, these white fibers are the ones that power lifters often tap into. Why? Because they activate when you're lifting super heavy weights for short durations like those powerlifting champs hoisting colossal barbells. These white fibers are like the muscle version of a turbocharged engine — they deliver incredible strength but are not too concerned about getting all pumped up and bulging.

And that's where the puzzle comes in. Power lifters can be incredibly strong, like the Hulk-strong, but they sometimes look like bodybuilders with those massive, chiseled muscles. Why? Because their training style primarily taps into those white fibers, which are all about brute strength, not bulking up. They're the masters of short, explosive bursts of power, but they're not into the whole "pumping iron" scene for hours.

On the flip side, bodybuilders are all about sculpting those show-stopping muscles, so they target the red fibers, especially the red slow-twitch ones. They're doing those countless reps and sets, pushing their powers to the limit and chasing that muscle pump like a golden ticket. That's why they end up with those massive, well-defined muscles — they're all about the "muscle hypertrophy" game.

But here's the kicker — there's much more to muscle growth than just which fibers you activate.

Things like nutrition, rest, genetics, and even hormones play roles in this muscle-building circus. And the truth is, you can train your muscles to be strong, like a power lifter, or big and chiseled, like a bodybuilder, depending on your goals and how you work those muscle fibers.

So, the next time you see a power lifter hoisting a barbell that looks like it could crush a small car, remember, they might not be going for the Arnold Schwarzenegger look – they're all about unleashing the power of those sneaky white fibers. Whether you're chasing strength, size, or both, remember, it's all about finding the right balance and pumping up those muscles to suit your fitness goals. It's like sculpting a work of art – you can choose your masterpiece!

***

Sweat and steam can do its job, but without a smart workout plan you won't be gaining much! Precisely the reason why you'll find many enthusiasts not having their desired arm gains despite all the added hours and sweat at the gym – pumping iron is one part of the gaining process but that's not all, the process, science and intellect involved in getting to the gain goals are equally critical. Let's dive into some secrets to sculpting those muscles into the masterpieces you've always envisioned.

- **Balance is Key**: You've pointed out the classic case of arm enthusiasts obsessing over biceps while neglecting the triceps. Remember, those triceps make up a whopping two-thirds of your arm size. If you want those arms to pop, it's essential to give both muscle groups equal attention. Balance your workouts to target all aspects of the muscle – that's how you achieve those symmetrical and awe-inspiring results.

• **Embrace the 3-Day Rule**: The muscle-building game is like a well-choreographed dance, and recovery is a crucial part of the performance. Muscles need approximately three days to repair and grow after a workout. If you're hammering the same muscle group day in and day out, you're not giving it the chance to rebuild properly. In fact, you might just be tearing down the same tissue over and over again – a classic case of spinning your wheels instead of making progress.

• **Variety is the Spice of Gains**: Don't get stuck in a workout rut. Mix it up! Change your exercises, angles, and intensity levels regularly. This not only prevents boredom but also keeps your muscles guessing, forcing them to adapt and grow. Muscles are like curious students; they thrive on new challenges.

• **Fuel Your Gains**: Nutrition is the foundation of muscle growth. Make sure you're getting enough protein to provide your muscles with the building blocks they need. Quality carbs and healthy fats are also essential for energy and overall health.

Hydration is often underestimated but plays a significant role in muscle function and recovery.

• **Rest like a Champ**: Don't underestimate the power of rest. It's during those precious hours of sleep that your body does most of its repair and growth work. Aim for 7-9 hours of quality shut-eye each night to maximize your gains.

• **Listen to Your Body**: Pay attention to how your body feels. If you're constantly sore, fatigued, or experiencing joint pain, it might be time to adjust your workout routine. Overtraining can lead to injuries and stall your progress.

• **Progressive Overload**: To keep those muscles growing, gradually increase the intensity of your workouts. This can be done by adding weight, increasing repetitions, or challenging yourself with advanced exercises. The name of the game is "progress."

So there you have it – the secrets to optimizing your muscle-building potential. It's all about finding the right balance, giving your muscles the time they need to recover, and keeping things fresh and exciting in the gym. Remember, Rome wasn't built in a day, and neither are your muscles. But with the right strategy and a sprinkle of patience, you'll be well on your way to achieving the physique you've been working hard for.

Don't let anyone tell you, "you're too skinny or fat to gain muscle." Use their negative energy against them because there is nothing further from the truth. Use it as fuel in the gym! It always feels good to prove people wrong. Be proud of yourself. Life is too short to care for the naysayers!

2 SHEDDING POUNDS, GAINING CONFIDENCE

Have you been fat-shamed lately? Have you been called names because you're overweight? That's bad! No one should have to go through such bullying – But why don't we get something positive out of this hurtful instance? It's time to embark on a transformative journey toward a healthier, more confident you. We now delve into the intricate landscape of fat loss with an unwavering commitment to nurturing your enthusiasm for the endeavor. As we proceed, we shall unravel the secrets to achieving a leaner physique while maintaining the ardor that ignited your passion for this noble pursuit.

But before we move on, you should know a little

something! The chapters come with a summative start, and then you'll have a roadmap to cut down the extra fats, followed by getting some.

The Pursuit of Fat Loss: A Journey of Inspiration

Consider your pursuit of fat loss as an epic odyssey—an adventure replete with challenges, triumphs, and profound personal growth. You are the hero in this narrative, embarking on a noble quest to unveil your latent potential. Each dietary choice each physical exertion, is a resolute stride towards self-discovery and transformation. So, ready yourself, for the voyage that lies ahead demands your unwavering resolve and perseverance.

Charting the Course for Success

In any monumental expedition, a meticulously planned route is essential for success. Your path to triumphant fat loss is no exception, and it is charted thus:

1. The Influential Role of Nutrition: Envision your body as a high-caliber instrument, akin to a meticulously tuned sports car. To propel your journey, it necessitates the finest fuel. Therefore, consume balanced meals emphasizing whole, unprocessed foods—vibrantly colored fruits and vegetables, lean proteins, and virtuous fats. Hydration must not be neglected, for water shall be your loyal companion on this trek.

2. Exercise as Your Arsenal: Regard your workouts

as the arsenal at your disposal—the most potent weapon in your quest for fat loss. Infuse variety into your regimen with strength training, cardiovascular exercise, and flexibility routines. This diversity not only augments fat loss but also preserves enthusiasm and engagement. Remember, a well-executed workout is not merely a physical exertion but an opportunity for rejuvenation and empowerment.

3. The Reverence of Rest and Recovery: Dismiss not the significance of a restful slumber. In the realm of fitness, sleep is akin to a mystical elixir—a transformative potion that heals and revitalizes your body. Cherish its restorative powers and honor it as an indispensable facet of your journey.

4. Cultivating an Indomitable Mindset: Throughout every noble quest, trials, and tribulations are bound to surface. Your mindset is the armor that shall shield you from adversity. Embrace positivity and resilience as your guiding principles. In your narrative, setbacks are a pivotal plot twist, never the denouement.

The Quest for Sustainable Fat Loss

In a fitness realm rife with ephemeral promises and fleeting solutions, we distinguish ourselves by pursuing sustainable fat loss—a transformation that transcends a mere phase, endures through a lifetime, and inspires perpetual self-assurance.

As you embark on this compelling expedition toward fat loss and newfound confidence, ponder this truth: each stride is a step closer to your aspirations. Every nourishing repast, every bead of sweat, and each affirmative thought brings you closer to the hero that destiny has ordained.

With your gear ready, your fervor ablaze, and your compass pointing steadfastly toward the realm of fat loss, we venture forth. In the forthcoming chapter, we shall delve into strategies designed to keep your motivation unwavering and to confront the inescapable roadblocks with grace and determination.

***

Pumped up already? Yeah! That's the spirit. Fat loss requires persistence and following a stringent fitness regime. I have figured out a generic roadmap, one that will fit anyone; from beginners to those who've already run the first mile, you could choose it to transform your weight loss goals. Obviously with expert and in-person help you can modify it as fitness is no one size fits all scheme. Let's begin!

1. The Inaugural Step: Consultation with a Healthcare Professional

Your weight loss journey begins with prudence. Seek counsel from a healthcare professional who can provide insights tailored to your unique health status and objectives. Their guidance will serve as the compass that steers us in the right direction.

2. Setting Sail with Clear Goals

Dreams transform into reality when they're well-defined. Here, we'll delve into the art of setting SMART goals—Specific, Measurable, Achievable, Relevant, and Time-bound. These goals will be the North Star guiding your voyage.

3. Navigating the Waters of Nutrition

Your journey is fueled by what you consume. Let's explore the intricacies of nutrition. However, details will come in the chapters to follow:

• Calculating your daily caloric needs and creating a sustainable calorie deficit for fat loss.

• Embracing whole, unprocessed foods rich in lean proteins, vibrant vegetables, wholesome grains, and healthy fats.

• Practicing mindful portion control and staying adequately hydrated.

4. Supplements: Allies on Your Quest

Supplements, like trusted companions, can support your journey.

• We'll unveil the secrets behind supplements such as protein powder, omega-3 fatty acids, multivitamins, creatine, and caffeine later as you read along. However, always consult with a healthcare professional before introducing supplements.

5. The Art of Sculpting: Exercise Regimens

Sculpting your physique is akin to crafting a masterpiece. Our exercise regimen comprises:

• Cardiovascular Workouts: Your cardiovascular health is paramount. Aim for 150 minutes of moderate-intensity aerobic exercise or 75 minutes of vigorous-intensity aerobic activity each week.

• Strength Training: We'll uncover the power of resistance workouts, emphasizing compound movements for strength and lean muscle.

• Flexibility Exercises: Improve mobility and reduce the risk of injury through stretching or yoga.

6. Rest, Rejuvenate, Repeat

• Your body's restoration is essential. Prioritize quality sleep—7-9 hours of rejuvenating slumber each night.

• Rest days in your training schedule are your body's oasis, preventing overtraining and facilitating muscle repair.

7. Progress Monitoring and Adaptation

• Regular progress checks are essential.

• Monitor metrics like body measurements, weight, body fat percentage, and strength gains.

• Flexibility and adaptability will be your allies, allowing you to make necessary adjustments along the way.

8. Wisdom from the Experts

• Utilize the wisdom of certified personal trainers or fitness coaches to design a personalized workout plan.

• For ongoing nutritional guidance and adjustments, seek counsel from registered dietitians.

9. Consistency as Your Steadfast Companion

• This journey is a marathon, not a sprint.

• Consistency and patience are your

companions, propelling you forward toward your goals.

10. The Mindset of a Champion

It's all in the mind, folks! You consider workout and diet a tedious task and start questioning your progress in the first week; you, my friend, are in for a loss! A positive mindset may be the last step, but is integral to your weight loss success.

Set your goals right and then stick to them – turn a deaf ear to the negativity, whatever the comments and catcalling be. It was there before when you weren't working out; it is here now that you've started improving your lifestyle, and believe it or not, the criticism will always be there. Rise beyond it and let your transformation do the magic of shutting it up. Considering the essential role of a transformational mindset that remains unmarred by its surrounding is focused on the results only I have dedicated an entire section that nurtures the athlete and fortifies the mind to keep hustling until the fats gone and you have your dream physique.

***

Your journey isn't just to transform your external appearance; it's an opportunity to unearth your inner athlete—a transformation that transcends appearances and revitalizes your entire outlook on life.

The first step in your transformation journey is cultivating the mindset that fuels it. This is more than just a quest to lose weight; it's a path to redefining yourself. Begin by reimagining who you are. Shed the identity of your past and envision the athlete you aspire to be—strong, capable, and resilient.

Embrace the process itself. Understand that this transformation isn't an instant revelation; it's a series of daily commitments and choices that collectively shape your future. Cherish each workout and each nutritious meal as a step toward the athlete you're becoming. Celebrate even the most minor achievements, for they are the building blocks of a better you.

Now, let's delve into the heart of your transformation—the thrilling journey of discovering your inner athlete:

• Start by defining your athletic identity. Picture the athlete you want to be: a runner, a weightlifter, a martial artist, or perhaps something entirely unique to you. Your athletic identity will serve as a guiding star, helping you make decisions aligned with your vision.

• Set concrete athletic goals. Do you dream of running a marathon, lifting a specific weight, or mastering a particular skill? Setting athletic goals that excite you will provide a sense of purpose and direction on your journey.

• Embrace your competitive spirit. Not to outdo others but to challenge yourself to become better than you were yesterday. Your greatest competition is your former self.

- Rediscover the joy in movement. Exercise isn't a form of punishment; it's a celebration of your body's capabilities. Try various formats of physical activity until you find one that ignites your passion and fills you with joy.

- Maintain consistency and patience. Transformations take time. Your unwavering commitment to the process and patience with your progress are your greatest allies.

- Seek inspiration in the stories of fellow athletes who've conquered challenges. Let their journeys fuel your determination and remind you that transformation is within your reach.

- Embrace discomfort and challenges as opportunities for growth. True transformation often occurs when you step outside your comfort zone.

- As you embark on this journey of fat loss and self-discovery, remember that the changes you're making extend far beyond the physical realm. This isn't merely about shedding pounds; it's about unearthing the athlete within, finding your inner strength, and redefining your entire perspective on life.

Imagine waking up each day with purpose, eager to pursue your athletic goals. Envision the boundless confidence from knowing you possess the inner resilience to conquer any obstacle. Your transformation isn't limited to your body; it encompasses your entire life.

In the following chapters, we'll delve deeper into the practical aspects of your transformation. From tailored workouts to nutritional strategies, we'll provide the tools to bring forth your inner athlete. Nevertheless, always remember that your change commences in your heart and mind. Embrace, nurture, and let it propel you toward the athlete you were destined to become.

"If you want and excuse you can always find one."
Elmer Bench (Breaking Bars Gym) Manning, SC

3 WORKOUTS THAT WORK WONDERS

So, imagine you've got your own fitness goals, just like I do. Your objectives really set the tone for the workout routine you choose. Our body, it's like this intricate machine that I can program, and it all starts with the health and fitness goals we set.

I mean, think about it, our brain is like the control center, sending signals to every cell, making sure they're all on the same page, working together to achieve my set goals. If my main aim is to lose fat, trust me, my body will react differently to a specific workout plan compared to someone who's not just targeting fat loss but also wants to gain muscle. It's like fitness goals are the big mission statement, and the workout regime is the detailed code that, when executed correctly, can turn me into super-fit software. Isn't it fascinating how we're all a bit like computers, just a tad more adaptable?

But let's not get lost in the philosophical weeds. Let's get back to the good stuff: various workout routines and what they can do for me and others like me – whether I'm an athlete, a fitness enthusiast, a beach body seeker, or even dreaming of building Herculean strength. So, let's break down some tried-and-tested workouts and see how they can help me and people with similar fitness dreams.

1. High-Intensity Interval Training (HIIT):

• Objectives: Elicit an acute metabolic response, promote lean body mass preservation, and enhance cardiovascular conditioning.

• Advantages: Induce post-exercise oxygen consumption, bolster cardiovascular resilience, and facilitate efficient calorie expenditure.

2. Strength Training:

• Objectives: Cultivate maximal force production, stimulate hypertrophy, and optimize body composition.

• Advantages: Foster increased neuromuscular coordination, elevate basal metabolic rate, and augment lean muscle accrual.

3. Cardiovascular/Aerobic Exercise:

• Objectives: Elevate VO2 max, enhance aerobic capacity, and promote calorie expenditure.

• Advantages: Boost myocardial efficiency, augment mitochondrial density, and facilitate body fat reduction.

4. **Yoga:**

• Objectives: Cultivate flexibility, enhance proprioception, and mitigate stress via mindfulness.

• Advantages: Bolster joint range of motion, improve somatosensory awareness, and ameliorate psychological well-being.

5. **Pilates:**

• Objectives: Strengthen the deep musculature, optimize core stability, and promote flexibility.

• Advantages: Cultivate lumbo-pelvic control, enhance postural alignment, and fortify the intrinsic muscle groups.

6. **Cross Fit:**

• Objectives: Emphasize functional fitness, encourage skill diversification, and nurture all-around athleticism.

• Advantages: Amplify metabolic conditioning, optimize work capacity, and bolster sport-specific competency.

7. **Circuit Training:**

• Objectives: Fuse resistance and cardiovascular exercises to enhance muscular endurance, cardiovascular fitness, and calorie expenditure.

• Advantages: Foster balanced physiological adaptation, amplify metabolic rate, and streamline workout efficiency.

8. Calisthenics:

• Objectives: Master Bodyweight movements to boost strength, proprioception, and agility.

• Advantages: Cultivate bodily control, augment relative strength, and stimulate lean muscle development.

9. Hiking and Trail Running:

• Objectives: Improve cardiovascular fitness, cultivate lower body endurance, and revel in the rejuvenating outdoors.

• Advantages: Elevate aerobic capacity, enhance lower extremity strength, and embrace the restorative power of nature.

10. Martial Arts:

• Objectives: Hone self-defense skills, refine martial techniques, and foster discipline and mental acuity.

• Advantages: Enhance combat readiness, instill focus and self-control, and attain an elevated level of physical and mental resilience.

Each fitness regimen presents a structured pathway to attaining specific physiological and performance objectives while offering a distinct array of benefits tailored to individual preferences and goals. Now that you know your preferred workout regime, let's delve into details of each workout.

***

High-Intensity Interval Training (HIIT) - The Fast Track to Fitness Excellence

In the quest for a leaner, stronger, and more resilient body, we encounter various workout regimes. However, none quite match the effectiveness and efficiency of High-Intensity Interval Training, more commonly known as HIIT. This chapter serves as your comprehensive guide to understanding the science, techniques, exercises, and dietary considerations that make HIIT a standout in the world of fitness.

The Science behind HIIT

HIIT isn't just another fitness trend; it's a well-established training methodology supported by science. At its core, HIIT involves alternating short bursts of high-intensity exercise with brief recovery periods. This approach triggers a cascade of physiological responses that yield exceptional results.

The acute metabolic response elicited by HIIT is a key factor. These intense intervals create a substantial oxygen debt that the body must repay post-workout. This repayment process results in the burning of additional calories, even when at rest. In other words, HIIT keeps your metabolic furnace roaring long after your workout ends, making it an efficient fat-burning strategy.

Furthermore, HIIT has been shown to preserve lean body mass. Unlike traditional steady-state cardio, which can lead to muscle loss, HIIT workouts protect your hard-earned muscle while helping you shed unwanted fat. This makes it a potent tool for achieving that toned and sculpted physique.

Cardiovascular conditioning is another standout feature of HIIT. By challenging your heart and lungs with intense bursts of activity, you improve your cardiovascular resilience and endurance. HIIT is like a high-intensity boot camp for your cardiovascular system, ensuring it performs at its best.

HIIT Exercises: A Dynamic Mix

A HIIT session is only as good as the exercises it comprises. Here's a lineup of some powerhouse moves to consider including in your HIIT routine:

• **Burpees**: A full-body exercise that engages multiple muscle groups simultaneously. It's fantastic for building strength and torching calories.

• **Mountain Climbers**: These keep your heart rate soaring and target your core muscles, providing a potent cardio and ab workout.

• **Jumping Jacks**: A classic move that works on your legs and arms, offering an excellent way to spike your heart rate.

• **Squats**: Ideal for sculpting your lower body, squats are essential for strong glutes and thighs.

• **Push-Ups**: The ultimate upper body workout, push-ups build chest, shoulder, and arm strength.

• **Sprints**: A straightforward yet highly effective form of HIIT, sprinting can be done on a track, a treadmill, or even outdoors. It's a tremendous calorie burner.

Fueling Your HIIT Journey

While the exercises are a crucial component of your HIIT routine, nutrition plays an equally vital role in your success. Here are some dietary considerations to keep in mind:

• **Protein**: Incorporate lean proteins like chicken, fish, and legumes into your diet. Protein supports muscle repair and growth, crucial for HIIT enthusiasts.

• **Complex Carbohydrates**: Whole grains, fruits, and vegetables provide sustained energy levels, helping you power through those intense intervals.

• **Healthy Fats**: Nuts, avocados, and olive oil are rich sources of healthy fats that support overall health and vitality.

• Hydration: Proper hydration is essential for peak performance. Ensure you drink adequate water before, during, and after your HIIT sessions.

• **Post-Workout Nutrition**: After your workout, opt for a protein-rich snack to aid in muscle recovery and repair.

In conclusion, High-Intensity Interval Training is a dynamic and scientifically-proven approach to fitness. Its unique ability to elevate metabolism, preserve muscle mass, and enhance cardiovascular fitness makes it a standout choice for individuals seeking efficient and effective workouts. When coupled with a balanced diet, HIIT becomes a potent tool in achieving your fitness goals, whether they involve fat loss, muscle gain, or improved overall conditioning. So, lace up your sneakers, embrace the intensity, and unlock the full potential of HIIT on your journey to fitness excellence.

***

Strength Training - Forging a Powerful Physique

Strength training, often referred to as resistance training or weightlifting, is the cornerstone of any comprehensive fitness program. It is the art and science of cultivating maximal force production, stimulating hypertrophy (muscle growth), and optimizing body composition. In this chapter, we delve into the profound benefits and proven methodologies of strength training, providing you with the knowledge and tools necessary to embark on your journey to a stronger, leaner, and healthier you.

The Science of Strength Training

Strength training is firmly rooted in scientific principles that govern the adaptation of the human body to resistance. At its core, it involves performing exercises that challenge muscles to overcome resistance, whether through free weights, machines, resistance bands, or body weight. This deliberate effort to challenge muscles beyond their accustomed limits leads to a range of physiological adaptations.

One of the primary objectives of strength training

is to stimulate muscle hypertrophy. Hypertrophy refers to the increase in muscle fiber size, and it is achieved by subjecting muscle groups to progressively heavier loads. As muscle fibers adapt to this stress, they become thicker and stronger, resulting in increased muscle mass and power.

Furthermore, strength training enhances neuromuscular coordination. This is the improved communication between the nervous system and muscle fibers, allowing for more efficient and synchronized muscle contractions. As a result, not only can you lift heavier weights, but you also perform daily activities with greater ease and grace.

The Advantages of Strength Training

Strength training bestows numerous advantages upon those who embrace it as a central component of their fitness routine:

• **Increased Basal Metabolic Rate (BMR)**: Muscle tissue is metabolically active, meaning it burns calories even at rest. By increasing muscle mass through strength training, you elevate your BMR, making it easier to maintain or lose weight.

• **Lean Muscle Accrual**: Strength training promotes the development of lean muscle mass while simultaneously reducing body fat percentage. This optimal body composition leads to a more sculpted and toned physique.

• **Improved Bone Density**: Resistance training is an effective means of enhancing bone density, reducing the risk of osteoporosis and fractures.

• **Enhanced Functional Strength**: The benefits of strength extend beyond the gym. Daily activities become more manageable, and the risk of injury during physical tasks decreases.

• **Disease Prevention**: Strength training has been linked to a lower risk of chronic conditions such as heart disease, diabetes, and arthritis.

Designing Your Strength Training Program

A well-structured strength training program is essential for achieving your fitness goals safely and effectively. Key elements of such a program include:

• **Exercise Selection**: Choose compound exercises that work multiple muscle groups simultaneously, such as squats, deadlifts, bench presses, and pull-ups.

• **Progressive Overload**: Gradually increase the resistance or intensity of your workouts to continually challenge your muscles and stimulate growth.

• **Repetition and Set Schemes**: Determine the number of sets and repetitions based on your objectives. For hypertrophy, moderate to high repetitions (8-12) are effective, while lower repetitions (1-6) are suitable for maximal strength development.

• **Rest Intervals**: Manage rest periods between sets to optimize recovery and performance.

• **Nutrition**: Support your strength training

efforts with a balanced diet that includes sufficient protein and overall caloric intake.

Backed by scientific research and proven methodologies, strength training is a powerful tool for achieving your fitness goals and enhancing your overall quality of life. As you embark on your strength training journey, remember that consistency, proper technique, and progressive overload are your allies in forging a stronger, healthier, and more resilient physique. So, with knowledge in hand, let's step into the weight room and unlock your full potential through the art and science of strength training.

***

Cardiovascular/Aerobic Exercise - Unleashing the Power of the Heart and Lungs

Cardiovascular or aerobic exercise is a fundamental component of any comprehensive fitness regimen, celebrated for its ability to elevate VO2 max (maximum oxygen uptake), enhance aerobic capacity, and promote calorie expenditure. In this chapter, we explore the science, benefits, and strategies behind cardiovascular training, providing you with a roadmap to harness the power of your heart and lungs for optimal health and fitness.

The Physiology of Cardiovascular Exercise

Cardiovascular exercise, often synonymous with

aerobic exercise, engages the body's cardiovascular and respiratory systems in an orchestrated effort to supply oxygen to working muscles and produce energy. When you engage in aerobic activities such as running, cycling, swimming, or brisk walking, your heart pumps more blood, delivering oxygen to muscles and removing waste products.

The primary objective of cardiovascular exercise is to improve VO2 max, a measure of the maximum amount of oxygen an individual can use during intense exercise. Elevating VO2 max signifies enhanced aerobic capacity, enabling you to sustain higher intensity levels for prolonged durations.

Advantages of Cardiovascular Exercise

• **Myocardial Efficiency**: Regular cardiovascular exercise improves the heart's efficiency in pumping blood, reducing the heart rate at rest and during exercise. This efficiency contributes to better cardiovascular health and overall endurance.

• **Mitochondrial Density**: Mitochondria are the energy powerhouses of cells. Cardiovascular exercise enhances mitochondrial density, improving the body's ability to utilize oxygen and produce energy during prolonged efforts.

• **Calorie Expenditure and Fat Reduction**: Aerobic workouts are potent calorie burners. By expending calories during exercise, coupled with an appropriate diet, cardiovascular exercise supports body fat reduction and weight management.

• **Improved Lung Function**: Aerobic activities enhance lung capacity and efficiency, ensuring an optimal exchange of oxygen and carbon dioxide during physical exertion.

Designing Your Cardiovascular/Aerobic Workout

To maximize the benefits of cardiovascular exercise, consider the following essential components:

• **Exercise Type**: Choose activities that elevate your heart rate and sustain it within your target heart rate zone for the desired duration. Options include running, cycling, swimming, brisk walking, and dancing.

• **Intensity**: Begin with moderate intensity and progress gradually to higher levels to challenge your cardiovascular system. Use tools like heart rate monitors to stay within your target heart rate zone.

• **Duration**: Aim for at least 150 minutes of moderate-intensity aerobic exercise per week, or 75 minutes of vigorous-intensity exercise, spread throughout the week.

• **Frequency**: Incorporate cardiovascular exercise into your routine at least 3-5 times per week for optimal results.

• **Rest and Recovery**: Allow your body adequate time to rest and recover between sessions to prevent overtraining and optimize performance.

By understanding the science behind cardiovascular exercise and applying proven training principles, you can harness the immense potential of your heart and lungs, leading to a healthier, fitter, and more energetic you.

***

Yoga - The Harmony of Body and Mind

Roots that have been dated back to more than five millennium, Yoga stands its place as one of the oldest and amongst the most potent fitness regime of all time. With its objectives rooted in cultivating flexibility, enhancing proprioception (the sense of one's body in space), and mitigating stress through mindfulness, yoga offers a holistic approach to physical and mental well-being. We delve into the profound science, myriad benefits, and the principles of yoga, providing you with a comprehensive understanding of this ancient practice's modern relevance.

The Alpha, Beta and Gamma of Yoga

Yoga, originating in ancient India, is a practice that harmonizes the body, mind, and spirit. At its core, yoga consists of physical postures (asanas), breath control (pranayama), and meditation. These elements work in concert to achieve a balanced state of physical and mental health.

One of yoga's primary objectives is to cultivate flexibility. Through a series of carefully designed postures, the body's range of motion is improved.

This flexibility enhances joint mobility, reduces the risk of injury, and contributes to overall physical resilience.

Additionally, yoga's emphasis on mindfulness and proprioception has been linked to reduced stress levels. The practice encourages heightened awareness of the present moment, fostering a sense of calm and mental clarity. This, in turn, contributes to the psychological well-being of practitioners.

The Advantages of Yoga

• **Joint Range of Motion**: Yoga postures systematically target various muscle groups and joints, increasing flexibility and promoting a greater range of motion. This is particularly beneficial for individuals seeking to alleviate stiffness and improve overall joint health.

• **Somatosensory Awareness**: Yoga encourages an enhanced sense of proprioception, or body awareness. Practitioners become attuned to the subtle movements and sensations within their bodies, improving balance and coordination.

• **Stress Mitigation**: Mindfulness and deep breathing techniques in yoga have been scientifically proven to reduce stress and anxiety. These practices enable individuals to manage the demands of modern life with greater ease and resilience.

• **Psychological Well-being**: Yoga's meditative aspects contribute to psychological well-being. Regular practice has been associated with improved mood, better emotional regulation, and increased self-awareness.

Designing Your Yoga Practice

Creating a fulfilling yoga practice requires thoughtful consideration of your objectives and preferences. Here are key components to keep in mind:

• **Yoga Styles**: Choose a style of yoga that aligns with your goals and comfort level. Hatha, Vinyasa, and Ashtanga are among the many yoga styles available, each offering unique characteristics and benefits.

• **Frequency**: Establish a regular practice routine. Whether it's daily or a few times a week, consistency is essential for reaping the benefits of yoga.

• **Guidance**: For beginners, attending classes led by experienced instructors can provide valuable guidance in terms of proper alignment and technique.

• **Home Practice**: As you progress, consider incorporating home practice sessions. Online resources and instructional videos are readily available to guide your practice.

• **Mindfulness**: Incorporate meditation and mindfulness exercises into your practice to harness the stress-reduction benefits of yoga fully.

Yoga is a profound practice that has withstood the test of time, offering a unique blend of physical and mental benefits. Its emphasis on flexibility, proprioception, and mindfulness allows practitioners to cultivate a harmonious relationship between body and mind. By embracing the principles of yoga and integrating them into your daily routine, you can unlock a path to enhanced well-being, reduced stress, and improved overall health.

***

CrossFit - A Holistic Fitness Revolution

Prepare to dive deep into the heart of CrossFit, a fitness phenomenon that marries scientific principles with real-world physical prowess. CrossFit's mission is nothing short of transforming ordinary individuals into well-rounded athletes, fostering functional fitness, skill diversification, and all-around athleticism. In this chapter, we embark on a journey through the science, methodologies, and multifaceted benefits of CrossFit, revealing the secrets of its remarkable success.

The CrossFit Science Spectrum

CrossFit's scientific underpinning stems from its fusion of weightlifting, gymnastics, and cardiovascular training. It represents an unyielding commitment to high-intensity, endlessly varied workouts that target not one, not two, but ten fitness domains: cardiovascular and respiratory endurance, stamina, strength, flexibility, power, speed, coordination, agility, balance, and accuracy. It's a fitness buffet designed to prepare you for the known and the unknown, a holistic approach that builds a resilient and capable body.

Advantages beyond Measure

Let's delve into the tangible advantages of CrossFit, which span the realms of metabolic conditioning, work capacity optimization, and sport-specific competency:

• **Metabolic Conditioning Marvel**: CrossFit turns up the metabolic heat. By pushing your body to the limit, it transforms you into a calorie-burning furnace. The result? Improved endurance, heightened stamina, and fat melting away.

• **Unleash Work Capacity**: CrossFit isn't just about working out; it's about working smarter. Through a blend of high-intensity routines, ever-changing movements, and minimal downtime, you'll find your work capacity skyrocketing.

• **Athlete in the Making**: CrossFit isn't just a workout; it's a lifestyle. Its diverse nature hones your skills and strengths, making you a well-rounded athlete ready to conquer various sports with newfound prowess.

Crafting Your CrossFit Experience

Now, let's talk about the art of crafting your CrossFit workouts, a canvas where fitness takes shape:

• **Warm-up**: Kick things off with a thorough warm-up that limbers up your body with mobility exercises and dynamic stretches, priming you for the challenges ahead.

• **Strength or Skill Component**: Weave strength training or skill-focused exercises into your routine to build specific movements and techniques.

• **The Heart of CrossFit - The WOD**: The Workout of the Day (WOD) is the centerpiece, a high-intensity medley that melds cardiovascular, weightlifting, and gymnastic elements into an exhilarating challenge.

• **Cool Down and Recovery**: Finally, let's not forget the cool-down phase. Stretch and foam roll to promote muscle recovery, ward off potential injuries, and bid adieu to those post-workout aches.

CrossFit is more than just exercise; it's a holistic approach to fitness that redefines your limits. By embracing its scientific principles, you'll unlock your work capacity, refine your metabolic conditioning, and bolster your athletic prowess. Step into the CrossFit arena, challenge your boundaries, and experience the transformative power of a fitness revolution that elevates you to new heights of physical excellence.

***

Maximizing Fitness Gains with Circuit Training

The Evolution of Circuit Training

Circuit training, initially gaining traction in the sports world during the mid-20th century, was devised to bolster both strength and endurance in athletes. Over time, it evolved beyond competitive sports, finding its place in mainstream fitness routines due to its ability to deliver a comprehensive workout experience.

At its core, circuit training thrives on efficiency. Incorporating various exercises into a structured circuit keeps the body in constant motion, elevating the heart rate. The circuit comprises several stations, each focusing on specific muscle groups or fitness goals. Participants move from one station to the next, engaging in exercises for a set duration or number of repetitions, often with minimal to no rest in between.

One of the most compelling aspects of circuit training is its adaptability. Whether you're a fitness newcomer or a seasoned athlete, circuit training can be tailored to meet your unique needs and preferences. The exercises can be customized based on your fitness level, available equipment, and specific fitness objectives, making it an inclusive workout suitable for diverse individuals.

Benefits That Resonate

Circuit training offers a multitude of benefits that resonate with fitness enthusiasts:

• **Efficient Time Utilization**: In today's fast-paced world, where time is of the essence, circuit training provides an efficient workout option. With minimal rest periods and continuous movement, it maximizes calorie burn and muscle engagement within a compact timeframe.

• **Strength and Endurance Boost**: Circuit training is a comprehensive workout, targeting different muscle groups to promote strength and endurance. The absence of extended rest periods enhances endurance and stamina, which is vital for athletes and everyday fitness enthusiasts alike.

• **Metabolic Activation**: Combining strength exercises and cardiovascular elements within a circuit ignites the metabolism. Even after the workout, calories burn, aiding in weight management and fat loss.

• **Sustained Engagement**: The various exercises and changing stations in a circuit keep the workout engaging, warding off monotony. This enhances physical benefits and maintains mental stimulation, fostering a commitment to the fitness routine.

• **Customizable for All Levels**: Circuit training's adaptability allows modifications to suit different fitness levels and accommodate varying physical capabilities. It accommodates all, regardless of their starting point, from bodyweight exercises to incorporating weights and resistance bands.

Crafting an Effective Circuit

Designing a robust circuit involves deliberate planning, considering the following aspects:

• **Exercise Selection**: Choose exercises that target diverse muscle groups, ensuring a well-rounded workout that combines compound and isolation movements.

• **Duration and Intensity**: Tailor the course or number of repetitions for each exercise, adjusting the intensity based on fitness level to maintain proper form and effectiveness.

• **Order and Flow**: Arrange exercises logically, considering muscle fatigue and alternating muscle groups for an efficient and smooth circuit flow.

• **Safety and Form**: Emphasize proper form and technique throughout the circuit to minimize injury risks. Encourage participants to listen to their bodies and make necessary adjustments for safety and effectiveness.

Dive into Circuit Training Exercises

Experience the circuit's power through a range of invigorating exercises:

• **Push-ups**: This fundamental exercise engages your chest, shoulders, and triceps.

• **Squats**: Target your quadriceps, hamstrings, and glutes, building lower body strength and endurance.

• **Jumping Jacks**: Elevate your heart rate, improving cardiovascular fitness and engaging multiple muscle groups.

• **Burpees**: Embark on a full-body challenge, activating legs, core, and arms for a high-intensity experience.

• **Plank**: Forge a rock-solid core while

strengthening your shoulders and gluteus, which is essential for overall stability.

• **Lunges**: Step forward to activate quadriceps, hamstrings, and glutes, refining lower body strength.

• **Dumbbell Rows**: Sculpt your back and biceps with precision using dumbbells.

• **Mountain Climbers**: Propel your heart rate and engage your core, enhancing cardiovascular endurance.

Fueling Your Circuit Journey with Nutrition

A well-balanced diet is a vital companion to your circuit training journey:

• **Balanced Macronutrients**: Maintain a harmonious balance of protein, carbohydrates, and healthy fats to support muscle recovery and sustain energy levels.

• **Hydration**: Stay adequately hydrated before, during, and after your workout to maintain performance and prevent dehydration.

• **Pre-Workout Nutrition**: Consume a balanced meal 2-3 hours before your workout, emphasizing complex carbohydrates and lean proteins.

• **Post-Workout Nutrition**: Within an hour post-workout, aim for a protein-rich meal or snack to aid muscle recovery and growth.

• **Healthy Snacking**: Incorporate wholesome snacks like nuts, fruits, and Greek yogurt to maintain energy levels throughout the day.

Embracing the Circuit Lifestyle beyond the

Workout

As you venture into the realm of circuit training, remember that your fitness journey encompasses more than just the circuit:

• **Rest and Recovery**: Adequate rest and recovery are pivotal for progress and injury prevention. Listen to your body's cues and allow for ample recovery between circuit training sessions.

• **Consistency**: The key to a successful fitness journey is unwavering consistency. Adhere to a regular circuit training schedule aligned with your fitness goals.

• **Guidance Matters**: Before commencing any new workout regimen or diet plan, consult a healthcare professional or certified trainer to ensure suitability for your needs and health status.

With these insights and a powerful arsenal of circuit training exercises, you're poised to sculpt a stronger, fitter version of yourself. Circuit training is not just a workout—it's a lifestyle, a journey towards a more vibrant and energetic you. Embark on this journey and let the circuits light your path to fitness excellence.

*****

Calisthenics: A Dive into Bodyweight Fitness Excellence

Have you explored the realm of calisthenics, an ancient fitness discipline rooted in Greek antiquity? The term 'calisthenics' stems from the fusion of 'kallos,' signifying beauty, and 'sthenos,' embodying strength. This amalgamation of aestheticism and physical prowess has not only stood the test of time but has also witnessed a contemporary resurgence due to its efficacy in fostering strength, flexibility, and a profound connection between body and mind.

In ancient Greece, calisthenics originated as a practice aligning beauty with strength, where individuals harnessed their body weight to achieve both. The concept evolved over centuries, influenced by various cultures and disciplines, eventually culminating in the holistic fitness approach we recognize today.

Core Tenets: Understanding Calisthenics' Essence

At its core, calisthenics leverages the resistance of one's own body weight to perform a diverse array of exercises. These exercises encompass a spectrum of movements, including pushing, pulling, bending, jumping, and swinging, engaging multiple muscle groups simultaneously. Calisthenics epitomizes the seamless fusion of artistry and strength in human movement.

Principles Underpinning Calisthenics

Let's delve into the foundational principles of calisthenics:

• **Bodyweight Resistance**: Calisthenics centers on utilizing one's body weight as the primary source of resistance, enabling muscle development and strength gains.

• **Progressive Overload**: The gradual increment of exercise difficulty ensures continual progress and muscle adaptation.

• **Controlled Movements**: Precise, controlled movements are pivotal in maintaining proper form and minimizing the risk of injury.

• **Full Range of Motion**: Complete range of motion in exercises is advocated to maximize muscle engagement and flexibility.

• **Mind-Body Connection**: Calisthenics emphasizes mindfulness and a strong mind-body connection.

The Perks of Calisthenics

Embarking on a calisthenics journey yields a host of benefits, including:

• **Strength and Muscle Development**: Calisthenics exercises target major muscle groups, promoting muscle growth and strength.

• **Flexibility and Mobility**: The dynamic movements in calisthenics enhance flexibility and mobility.

• **Functional Fitness**: Calisthenics emphasizes movements relevant to daily activities, enhancing functional fitness and overall performance.

• **Minimal Equipment Requirement**: Calisthenics is accessible, requiring little to no equipment.

• **Versatility and Scalability**: The adaptability

of calisthenics renders it suitable for individuals of all fitness levels.

Foundational Calisthenics Exercises

• **Push-ups**: Targets chest, shoulders, and triceps.

• **Pull-ups/Chin-ups**: Engages the back, biceps, and forearms.

• **Squats**: Targets the quadriceps, hamstrings, and glutes.

• **Plank**: Engages the core, shoulders, and glutes.

• **Dips**: Targets the triceps and chest.

• **Lunges**: Works the lower body, emphasizing the quadriceps and glutes.

Constructing an Effective Calisthenics Regimen

Crafting a well-rounded calisthenics routine involves:

• **Warm-up**: Initiating the workout with a dynamic warm-up prepares the body for exercise and prevents injury.

• **Skill Development**: Focusing on mastering specific exercises and improving technique is crucial for progress and efficacy.

• Strength Training: Incorporating various calisthenics exercises targeting different muscle groups forms the foundation of the workout.

• **Skill Progression**: Advancing to more challenging variations of exercises as strength improves is essential for continual growth and adaptation.

• **Cool Down and Stretching**: Concluding the workout with static stretching aids in flexibility and muscle recovery.

Nourishment and Recovery in Calisthenics

• **Balanced Diet**: Maintaining a balanced diet rich in protein, carbohydrates, healthy fats, vitamins, and minerals supports muscle recovery and growth.

• **Hydration**: Staying well-hydrated is crucial for performance and overall health.

• **Adequate Rest and Recovery**: Allowing muscles ample time to recover and repair after intense calisthenics sessions is essential for optimal performance and growth.

Calisthenics is more than just a fitness regimen; it's a testament to the human body's capabilities and an invitation to explore one's limits. Combining ancient wisdom and modern understanding makes calisthenics a profound and practical approach to holistic fitness. Embrace this journey, and let your body be a canvas for the art of strength. Happy training!

***

Martial Arts: Unveiling the Art of Discipline and Strength

Have you ever considered the profound world of martial arts? It's a captivating realm where the fusion of discipline, strength, and tradition elevates body and mind to exceptional levels. Let's embark on this exploration into the world of martial arts, where ancient practices meet modern understanding to create a holistic approach to physical and mental well-being.

As we delve into the ancient physically testing and mentally challenging martial arts, allow me to share my remarkable journey with you. I hold the esteemed rank of a black belt in Tang Soo Do, and my mastery extends to the revered Kenpo discipline. In the realm of Tae Kwon Do, I've attained the prestigious status of a fourth gup which is 3 belts lower than black belt. Additionally, my journey in Brazilian Jiu-Jitsu has led me to the coveted blue belt.

But here's where the story truly takes flight—a moment of triumph that defines my dedication and indomitable spirit. In the fiercely competitive arena of martial arts, I took on the world in the 2014 Tang Soo Do Championship. What makes this achievement truly extraordinary is the undeniable challenge I faced—a torn hamstring, an obstacle that would deter most.

Despite this formidable setback, I pushed forward with unwavering determination and resilience. My journey wasn't just about fighting opponents in the ring; it was a battle against adversity, a test of character, and a display of sheer willpower.

And the result? I clinched the remarkable 3rd place in the World Tang Soo Do Championship in sparring, a feat that echoes the relentless pursuit of excellence, even in the face of physical adversity. It's a testament to the human spirit's capacity to soar beyond its limits. All his endurance and will was multiplied by the intensive physical and mental training that's involved in this esteemed body art and training regime.

Coming back to the basics. Martial arts trace their roots back to ancient civilizations, where combat techniques were refined for self-defense and warfare. Over centuries, these practices evolved into formalized systems, incorporating philosophical and spiritual elements. From the battlefields of Asia to global dojos, martial arts have become a diverse and rich tapestry of traditions and styles.

At the core of martial arts lie fundamental principles that extend beyond physical combat. Concepts such as respect, discipline, humility, and perseverance are central. The mental and spiritual aspects are as crucial as the physical techniques, fostering a harmonious balance within practitioners.

Diverse Styles and Techniques

Martial arts encompass a vast array of styles, each with its unique techniques and philosophies. Some types emphasize striking techniques, while others focus on grappling or combining both. From Karate's powerful strikes to the grace of Kung Fu and the discipline of Brazilian Jiu-Jitsu, there's a style to suit every individual.

Benefits of Martial Arts Practice

Engaging in martial arts offers a multitude of benefits, including:

• **Physical Fitness**: Martial arts enhance strength, flexibility, coordination, and cardiovascular health. Training involves a variety of exercises that challenge the entire body.

• **Self-Defense Skills**: Learning martial arts equips individuals with valuable self-defense techniques, boosting confidence and personal safety.

• **Stress Reduction**: The meditative and focused nature of martial arts practice helps reduce stress and improve mental well-being.

• **Character Development**: Martial arts instill values such as discipline, respect, perseverance, and self-control, fostering positive character development.

• **Community and Camaraderie**: Training in martial arts often involves a tight-knit community, providing social interaction and support.

Martial Arts Training: The Journey of a Martial Artist

The journey of a martial artist is one of dedication and continuous learning. It involves progressive levels of training, often represented by colored belts and the pursuit of mastery through diligent practice and guidance from experienced instructors.

Ensuring the safety and well-being of practitioners is paramount in martial arts. Ethical conduct, respect for opponents, and proper training techniques are fundamental to a positive martial arts experience.

Embracing the Martial Arts Lifestyle

Martial arts is not merely a physical practice; it's a way of life. Beyond the dojo, the principles and philosophies of martial arts can be applied to everyday life, promoting mindfulness, discipline, and respect in all endeavors.

Martial arts is not limited to combat skills. They encompass a holistic approach to life, nurturing the body and mind. So, whether you're drawn to the grace of Aikido, the power of Muay Thai, or the discipline of Taekwondo, stepping onto the martial arts path is a journey toward self-discovery, resilience, and empowerment.

***

You could be Kung-Fu, master or a marathon runner, fitness comes with consistency and proper goal setting. Scheduling your workout remains essential as no two muscles could be trained every day and expect returns over them. In my fitness journey, I've found that a 2-days-on and 1-day-off split works exceptionally well for optimizing muscle building and fat loss. This tailored routine is designed to ensure every muscle group gets attention while allowing adequate recovery. I won't want you to strictly adhere to this only, you could obviously customize it or find something new as well, but if you want something tried and tested, here it is:

On day one, I focus on chest and triceps. Pushing

exercises primarily engage the chest, and by extending the workout to include triceps, I'm maximizing muscle engagement and growth.

Day two revolves around back and biceps. Pulling exercises engage the back muscles, and incorporating bicep exercises on this day complements the workout, given their involvement in pulling movements.

A well-deserved rest on day three allows my body to recover and prepare for the next round of training.

Day four is dedicated to working the lower body—legs. Incorporating squats, lunges, and other leg exercises ensures a comprehensive lower body workout, promoting strength and muscle growth.

Day five targets shoulders, an area often overlooked. Well-developed shoulders not only complete the aesthetic physique but also contribute to overall upper body strength.

After this workout cycle, a day of rest is essential before diving back into the routine. This split not only optimizes muscle building and fat loss but also allows for the necessary recovery to prevent overtraining. So, what I think is; Once you've set the goal, selected your preferred workout regime, it all comes down to consistency and scheduling your exercises, following diet and being patient! Towards the end of this extremely informative episode in our journey towards a stronger, fitter and healthier you, always know that:

Try not to laugh if you see someone doing an exercise that you think looks ridiculous. Maybe they have a goal or mechanical disadvantage that you don't know about.

4 DIVE INTO DIETS: FROM KETO TO KETTLEBELLS

The Keto-Kettlebell Connection. We're talking about how food and fitness come together to make you feel like a superhero in your own life. While name might depict something that only concerns Keto diet and Kettlebell workout, on the contrary it aims to take you into a bigger world where diet and workout come together to make a superb physique.

So, here's the deal: Keto. It's not your usual diet where you're counting calories or eating tiny salads. No, sir. This is a wild ride where you kick carbs to the curb and welcome fats to the party. The goal? Get your body to burn fat for fuel instead of carbs. Sounds like science fiction, but it's the real deal.

But hold your horses! Before you jump headfirst into the Keto adventure, know this: it's not all bacon and avocados. You've got to be smart about it. It's about finding a balance, so you don't miss out on important stuff. And hey, be ready for the keto flu. Your body's way of saying, "Hey, what's going on here?" It might be a little bumpy, but trust me, the destination is worth the ride.

Now, let's switch gears to kettlebells. We're not just talking about lifting weights here; we're talking about these cannonball-like weights that bring a whole new meaning to the word 'versatile.' With kettlebells, you've got a full-body workout at your fingertips. Swings, snatches, Turkish get-ups - it's like a fitness adventure park in one piece of equipment. Plus, it's super time-efficient, which is great for those of us with busy schedules.

But, and this is a big 'but,' you can't just grab a kettlebell and start swinging it around like a wild cowboy. Technique matters, my friends. It's not a free-for-all; it's an art form. So, start with someone who knows the ropes. An instructor or a beginner's program - they're your safety net.

Now, let's put it all together. Keto and kettlebell training, they're like peanut butter and jelly. Each complements the other. But here's the secret sauce: you need a coach, a mentor, to guide you. Before you set off on this wild adventure, let's chat about your goals, your health, and your own unique roadmap.

This journey into the world of Keto and Kettlebells is like an epic quest, while we are already through the workout regimes it's time we hit the diet and food bay! So, what do you say we get this show on the road?

***

You know, when it comes to getting fit and carving out that dream physique, diet is where the magic happens. It's like the secret ingredient to the whole fitness recipe. What we put in our bodies has a massive say in how we look and feel. So, welcome to our diet adventure. We're about to explore an exciting menu of diets, each tailored for specific fitness and physique goals.

From beefing up those muscles with a high-protein diet to zapping fat with Keto's metabolic mojo and even finding Zen in plant-based nutrition, I've got it all sorted out for you. We're going to break down the goals, the perks, and what makes each diet unique. The goal here is to arm you with the knowledge you need to make the right dietary choices for your fitness journey. Let's get started!

1. High-Protein Diet:

Goal: Muscle Building and Repair

Advantages: A high-protein diet is essential for those looking to build and repair muscles. It provides the amino acids necessary for muscle growth and recovery. Protein also has a high thermic effect, which means it burns more calories during digestion, aiding in weight management.

2. Keto Diet (Ketogenic Diet):

Goal: Fat Loss and Improved Metabolism

Advantages: The Keto diet is designed to shift your body into a state of ketosis, where it primarily burns fat for fuel. This can lead to significant fat loss and improved metabolic health. Additionally, some individuals find increased mental clarity and sustained energy levels while on the Keto diet.

3. Balanced Macronutrient Diet:

Goal: Overall Fitness and Well-being

Advantages: A balanced diet, which includes a good mix of carbohydrates, proteins, and fats, is ideal for those who want to maintain a healthy weight, have sustained energy levels, and support overall fitness. It provides the nutrients needed for both physical activity and daily life.

4. Intermittent Fasting:

Goal: Weight Management and Insulin Sensitivity

Advantages: Intermittent fasting focuses on when you eat rather than what you eat. It can help regulate insulin sensitivity, promote fat loss, and improve body composition. It also simplifies meal planning for some individuals.

5. Plant-Based Diet:

Goal: Health, Weight Management, and Environment

Advantages: A plant-based diet primarily focuses

on whole foods from plants. It is rich in fiber, antioxidants, and various nutrients. It can support overall health, help with weight management, and is environmentally friendly. Additionally, it reduces the risk of chronic diseases.

6. Paleo Diet:
Goal: Whole Food Consumption and Reduced Inflammation

Advantages: The Paleo diet emphasizes whole, unprocessed foods, which can help reduce inflammation in the body. It is suitable for those who wish to maintain a natural, nutrient-dense diet that may aid in fitness and overall health.

7. Mediterranean Diet:
Goal: Heart Health and Longevity

Advantages: The Mediterranean diet is rich in heart-healthy fats, whole grains, lean proteins, and a variety of fruits and vegetables. It's associated with a reduced risk of heart disease and has anti-inflammatory and anti-aging benefits.

8. Low-Carb Diet:
Goal: Weight Loss and Blood Sugar Control

Advantages: Low-carb diets can promote weight loss by reducing insulin levels and increasing fat burning. They're beneficial for those seeking to manage blood sugar levels and improve overall metabolic health.

Fit for a different set of fitness goals and a totally different physique, each diet needs apt knowledge of your goals and your body's ability to consume and digest the food included. To learn this better read along for details of diet and choose wisely under the supervision of a certified nutritionist. Till then read along and learn more!

***

To keep it simple for you, I've sorted the type of diets with their potential advantages, timings and type of food intake so you may find them to help you best.

Let's go!

High-Protein Food Types

Ready to pump up the protein? These are your trusty allies for building and repairing those hard-earned muscles: lean meats like chicken and turkey, the mighty fish duo of salmon and tuna, eggs (nature's protein bombs), and dairy champs like Greek yogurt and cottage cheese. If you're into the plant-based vibe, tofu, lentils, and chickpeas have got your back. And don't forget the crunch – nuts and seeds like almonds and chia seeds bring protein power to your snacking game.

1. Optimal Timing for Protein Intake:

Breakfast Boost: Kickstart your metabolism with a protein-packed breakfast. Think scrambled eggs with veggies or a smoothie with protein powder.

Post-Workout Refuel: After crushing your workout, aim to refuel with protein within 2 hours. A protein shake or a chicken and quinoa bowl works wonders.

Snacks with Punch: Between meals, sneak in a protein-rich snack to keep hunger at bay. Greek yogurt with some berries or a handful of almonds should do the trick.

Dinner Delight: End the day with a dinner that's easy on your digestion but heavy on protein. Grilled chicken or a piece of salmon with veggies will support muscle maintenance as you sleep like a champ.

2. Benefits of a High-Protein Diet:

Muscle Magic: Protein is your muscle's best friend, helping them grow and recover after workouts.

Metabolic Makeover: It revs up your metabolism by burning more calories during digestion.

Weight Whiz: Protein helps control your appetite and may lead to better weight management.

Feeling Full: You'll feel full and satisfied, making it easier to resist those tempting snacks.

Fat Farewell: It might just be your secret weapon for burning that stubborn body fat.

3. High-Protein Diet Tips:

Stay Hydrated: Protein digestion needs water, so keep the H2O flowing.

Fiber Friends: Balance your protein intake with fiber-rich foods for a well-rounded diet.

Portion Patrol: Be mindful of portions – more protein doesn't mean more is always better.

Pro Help: If you're diving deep into a high-protein

journey, consider consulting a dietitian for personalized guidance.

4. Sample High-Protein Day:

Breakfast Bliss: Start your day with scrambled eggs and spinach, plus a slice of whole-grain toast.

Snack Attack: Keep it simple with Greek yogurt topped with berries and a drizzle of honey.

Lunch Love: Grilled chicken salad with a rainbow of veggies and a zesty vinaigrette – lunch done right.

Snack Time Again: A handful of almonds or a protein smoothie to keep your energy up.

Dinner Delight, Round 2: Wrap it up with baked salmon, a side of quinoa, and a heap of steamed broccoli.

***

Keto Diet (Ketogenic Diet)

1. Keto-Friendly Foods:

Get ready to dive into the world of Keto-approved foods:

Healthy fats (avocado, olive oil, nuts)

Fatty fish (salmon, mackerel)

Low-carb vegetables (spinach, cauliflower, zucchini)

Lean proteins (chicken, turkey)

Dairy (cheese, Greek yogurt)

2. Timing Your Keto Journey:

Morning Ketosis Kickstart: Start your day with a Keto-friendly breakfast, like an omelet with avocado.

Post-Workout Replenish: After a workout, opt for

a protein and healthy fat combo to help recovery.

Keto Snack Attack: Keep hunger at bay with snacks like nuts or a handful of berries.

Keto Dinner Delight: Make dinner shine with a fatty fish and low-carb veggies.

3. Advantages of the Keto Diet:

Fat Furnace: Keto shifts your body into fat-burning mode, leading to substantial fat loss.

Metabolic Marvel: It revs up your metabolism for better calorie burning.

Mental Clarity: Some folks find their focus and clarity skyrocket on Keto.

Steady Energy: Say goodbye to energy dips; Keto keeps you powered up.

4. Keto Tips and Tricks:

Hydration is Key: Keep up the water intake to support your body's new metabolism.

Mindful Macros: Track your carb intake, keeping it super low.

Balanced Plate: Ensure your meals are a mix of fats, proteins, and low-carb veggies.

Consult a Pro: If you're going deep into Keto, a dietitian can offer personalized guidance.

5. A Sample Keto Day:

Keto Morning: Start with an omelet loaded with veggies and some avocado.

Keto Snack: Enjoy a handful of almonds or some Greek yogurt.

Keto Lunch: Dive into a salad with chicken, plenty

of leafy greens, and a keto-friendly dressing.

Keto Snack Round 2: Keep the energy flowing with cheese and cucumber slices.

Keto Dinner: Indulge in baked salmon with a side of cauliflower mash.

***

Balanced Macronutrient Diet

1. A Palette of Macronutrients:

The beauty of this diet lies in balance, a culinary canvas filled with:

Carbohydrates (whole grains, fruits, vegetables)

Proteins (lean meats, beans, dairy)

Fats (avocado, nuts, olive oil)

2. Timing Your Balanced Journey:

Breakfast Brilliance: Start your day with a balanced meal of oats, Greek yogurt, and some fruit.

Lunchtime Harmony: A well-rounded salad with greens, lean protein, and a sprinkle of nuts is a winner.

Smart Snacking: Munch on some carrot sticks with hummus or a piece of string cheese between meals.

Dinner Delight: Close the day with a balanced plate featuring grilled chicken, quinoa, and roasted veggies.

3. Goals of the Balanced Macronutrient Diet:

All-Around Fitness: It's your passport to overall health and fitness.

Sustained Energy: Keeping you fueled throughout the day.

Nutrient Harmony: A diet that hits all the right nutritional notes.

Weight Wellness: Supporting healthy weight management.

4. Tips for a Balanced Diet:

Colorful Plate: Aim for variety and include a rainbow of fruits and vegetables.

Portion Power: Keep portion sizes in check to manage calorie intake.

Fiber Focus: Prioritize fiber-rich foods for digestion and fullness.

Seek Guidance: Consult a dietitian for personalized advice on meal planning.

5. A Sample Balanced Day:

Balanced Breakfast: A hearty breakfast with whole-grain toast, scrambled eggs, and some mixed berries.

Balanced Snack: Greek yogurt with a drizzle of honey keeps you going.

Balanced Lunch: A colorful salad with mixed greens, grilled chicken, and a vinaigrette dressing.

Balanced Snack Encore: Crunch on a handful of mixed nuts or a piece of fruit.

Balanced Dinner: Savor a dinner of baked salmon with brown rice and steamed broccoli.

***

Intermittent Fasting

1. The Art of Timing:

Intermittent fasting isn't so much about what you

eat but when you eat. It's divided into fasting periods and eating windows:

16/8 Method: 16 hours of fasting, 8 hours of eating.

5:2 Method: Five days of regular eating, two days of extreme calorie restriction.

Eat-Stop-Eat: Full-day fasts once or twice a week.

2. Timing Your Fasting Journey:

Morning Fast: Start your fasting period after dinner and skip breakfast.

Lunchtime Fast: Skip breakfast and wait until lunch to break your fast.

Early Dinner Fast: Conclude your eating early in the evening and have a late breakfast.

3. Goals of Intermittent Fasting:

Weight Wizardry: It's all about managing your weight.

Insulin Insights: Fasting can improve your body's sensitivity to insulin.

Metabolic Mastery: Boosting metabolism and enhancing fat burning.

Simplicity and Convenience: It simplifies your meal planning and timing.

4. Tips for Successful Intermittent Fasting:

Stay Hydrated: Drink water, herbal tea, or black coffee during fasting periods.

Choose Nutrient-Rich Foods: When you eat, focus on whole, nutrient-dense foods.

Listen to Your Body: If fasting doesn't suit you,

consider alternative approaches.

Consult a Professional: Before diving deep into fasting, discuss it with a healthcare provider.

5. A Sample Intermittent Fasting Day:

Fasting Window: From 8 PM to 12 PM (16-hour fast).

Breaking the Fast: A well-balanced lunch with lean protein, vegetables, and whole grains.

Afternoon Snack: A piece of fruit or a handful of nuts.

Dinner: A hearty meal with a focus on nutrients.

Closing the Eating Window: Finish your last meal by 8 PM.

***

Plant-Based Diet

1. A Feast of Plants:

The star of this dietary show? Plants, of course! Your plate will be brimming with:

Fruits and vegetables

Whole grains

Legumes (beans and lentils)

Nuts and seeds

Plant-based proteins (tofu, tempeh)

2. Plant-Powered Timing:

Morning Green Start: Begin your day with a green smoothie or a fruit-packed bowl.

Balanced Lunch: A hearty salad, veggie wrap, or plant-based soup.

Smart Snacking: Munch on a handful of nuts or

sliced veggies with hummus.

Dinner Delight: Cap it off with a plant-based protein (tofu or legumes), grains, and a generous helping of greens.

3. Goals of the Plant-Based Diet:

Health Hero: It's your ticket to overall health and well-being.

Weight Wellness: Supporting healthy weight management.

Eco-Warrior: You're making a positive impact on the environment.

Nutrient Abundance: Reaping the benefits of plant-derived nutrients.

4. Tips for Embracing a Plant-Based Lifestyle:

Variety is Vital: Embrace a rainbow of fruits and veggies.

Protein Prowess: Explore plant-based protein sources like tofu and legumes.

Whole Grains Galore: Opt for whole grains for a fiber boost.

Supplement Sensibly: Consider vitamin B12 and other key nutrients if needed.

5. A Sample Plant-Based Day:

Plant-Powered Breakfast: A smoothie with spinach, banana, and chia seeds.

Plant-Based Lunch: A quinoa and black bean salad with avocado.

Plant-Based Snack: Fresh fruit or a handful of

almonds.

Plant-Based Dinner: Stir-fried tofu with a medley of colorful veggies and brown rice.

***

Paleo Diet

1. The Caveman's Delight:

Welcome to the age of the caveman. Your menu features foods that our hunter-gatherer ancestors would've devoured:

Lean meats (grass-fed beef, poultry)

Fish

Fruits and vegetables

Nuts and seeds

Healthy fats (olive oil, coconut oil)

2. Paleo Planning:

Primordial Breakfast: Kickstart your day with a Paleo-friendly meal – perhaps scrambled eggs with veggies.

Lunch from the Past: A salad with grilled chicken, nuts, and olive oil dressing.

Ancient Snacking: Munch on some fresh fruit or a handful of almonds.

Dinner the Paleo Way: Savor a piece of grilled salmon, steamed veggies, and a side of sweet potato.

3. Goals of the Paleo Diet:

Whole Food Wonder: It's all about consuming unprocessed, natural foods.

Inflammation Buster: Aiding in reducing inflammation in your body.

Nourishing Nutrients: You're soaking up the goodness of whole foods.

Weight Wellness: Supporting healthy weight management.

4. Tips for Embracing the Paleo Lifestyle:

Ditch Processed Fare: Say goodbye to processed foods and sugar.

Quality Meats Matter: Opt for lean, grass-fed meats.

Fiber Focus: Load up on fruits, vegetables, and nuts for fiber.

Stay Hydrated: Water should be your beverage of choice.

5. A Sample Paleo Day:

Paleo Breakfast: A hearty omelet with spinach, tomatoes, and avocado.

Paleo Lunch: A generous salad with grilled chicken, nuts, and a drizzle of olive oil.

Paleo Snack: A piece of fresh fruit or a handful of almonds.

Paleo Dinner: Baked salmon with roasted veggies and sweet potato.

***

Mediterranean Diet

1. The Mediterranean Tapestry:

Welcome to the sun-kissed shores of the Mediterranean. Your plate is adorned with:

Heart-healthy fats (olive oil, nuts)

Lean proteins (fish, poultry)

Whole grains (whole wheat, brown rice)

Abundant fruits and vegetables

A sprinkle of herbs and spices

2. Mediterranean Menu Moments:

Sunrise by the Sea: Kick off the day with a whole-grain toast drizzled with olive oil and a side of fresh fruit.

Coastal Charm: A Mediterranean salad with greens, grilled fish, and a handful of nuts.

Between Meals Oasis: Sip on herbal tea or snack on fresh veggies with hummus.

Dinner Delights: Dive into a roasted chicken dish with a colorful medley of veggies and whole grains.

3. Goals of the Mediterranean Diet:

Heart Health Haven: It's your recipe for a happy heart and a longer life.

Anti-Inflammatory: Taming inflammation with nature's bounty.

Youthful Longevity: Enhancing your chances of a long, healthy life.

Culinary Bliss: Savoring the joys of Mediterranean cuisine.

4. Tips for Savoring the Mediterranean Lifestyle:

Olive Oil Obsession: Use olive oil as your primary source of fat.

Fish Fiesta: Incorporate fish, especially fatty fish, regularly.

Rainbow of Produce: Embrace the color and

variety of fruits and vegetables.

Mindful Meals: Savor your meals, ideally with family and friends.

5. A Sample Mediterranean Day:

Mediterranean Morning: Whole-grain toast with olive oil and a fruit salad.

Mediterranean Lunch: A Greek salad with feta, olives, and grilled salmon.

Mediterranean Snack: Sip on herbal tea or nibble on fresh veggies with hummus.

Mediterranean Dinner: Roasted chicken with a side of couscous and a garden salad.

***

Low-Carb Diet

1. Cutting the Carbs:

This diet is all about reducing carbohydrate intake, and your plate will feature:

Lean proteins (chicken, fish)

Non-starchy vegetables (leafy greens, broccoli)

Healthy fats (avocado, nuts)

Limited fruits

Minimal grains and sugar

2. Low-Carb Dining Delights:

Carb-Conscious Breakfast: Start the day with scrambled eggs, spinach, and a sprinkle of cheese.

Lean Lunch: A salad with grilled chicken and a balsamic vinaigrette.

Snack Smart: Nibble on almonds or veggie sticks with guacamole.

Dinner without Carbs: Savor a piece of grilled fish with steamed asparagus.

3. Goals of the Low-Carb Diet:

Weight Whittler: It's your tool for shedding pounds and managing your weight.

Blood Sugar Savvy: Helps control blood sugar levels and insulin sensitivity.

Appetite Awareness: Keeps your appetite in check.

Reduced Sugar Impact: Limits sugar and refined carbs.

4. Tips for Navigating a Low-Carb Lifestyle:

Quality Carbs: If you include carbs, prioritize whole grains and non-starchy veggies.

Protein Priority: Choose lean proteins for satiety.

Healthy Fats: Embrace avocados, nuts, and olive oil.

Hydration Help: Stay well-hydrated.

5. A Sample Low-Carb Day:

Low-Carb Breakfast: Scrambled eggs with sautéed spinach.

Low-Carb Lunch: A chicken Caesar salad without croutons.

Low-Carb Snack: Almonds or cucumber slices with guacamole.

Low-Carb Dinner: Grilled salmon with a side of steamed asparagus.

***

In my journey towards better health and fitness, I've embarked on two distinct dietary paths - the

"Bulking Up" and "Trimming Down" phases. Each carries its unique story and a valuable lesson for anyone on a similar quest.

During my "Bulking Up" phase, I become a relentless eater, embracing a feast of calories. It's not just about eating everything in sight, but rather about fulfilling a purpose - building muscle and strength. My daily mission? To consume a minimum of 1 gram of protein for each pound of my body weight. It's a formidable challenge that requires dedication and, well, a hearty appetite.

Now, in my "Trimming Down" phase, I turn to a low-glycemic carbohydrate diet. Here, the lessons revolve around restraint and selective choices. Fruit, despite its health benefits, is off the menu due to its sugar content. Lean cuts of beef, chicken breast, and fish become my protein allies. The carb category narrows down to brown rice, yams, and oatmeal. And my plate is an homage to green vegetables.

But here's the catch. No matter which path I tread, there are universal principles that should guide us all. It's a lesson in mindfulness. I've learned to scrutinize ingredient lists, keeping a vigilant eye out for sugar and sneaky culprits like malt dextrin. The beverages that accompany my meals are pure and simple - water and Crystal Light.

Through these dietary duality, I've come to realize that there's no one-size-fits-all approach to health and fitness. We're all on our unique journeys, and what works for one might not work for another. The key is to learn from our experiences, make informed choices, and find balance.

So, whether you're bulking up, trimming down, or simply looking to maintain a healthy lifestyle, the overarching lesson here is to listen to your body, do your research, and adapt your diet to suit your goals and preferences. Food isn't just fuel; it's a versatile tool that can be tailored to sculpt your best self.

Just because you see a ripped bodybuilder eating a fat juicy bacon cheeseburger doesn't mean you should. Remember that people have different metabolism and body goals. They may also be taking performance enhancing supplements.

5 STEROIDS: UNVEILING THE SCIENCE

In the dynamic world of bodybuilding and fitness, there exists a hidden narrative that has captivated both athletes and scientific minds for decades: steroids. These precisely engineered synthetic compounds, designed to mimic the anabolic prowess of endogenous hormones, have cast a substantial shadow across the landscape of competitive sports and physique enhancement.

As we strip away the layers of this 'secret catalyst', we find steroids rooted within the realm of bodybuilding for years. They are something that aren't new to fitness lovers, but a parcel of human attempts at hitting the superhuman aura for centuries. Born of curiosity and ambition, steroids have perennially been shrouded in controversy, with their origin stories deeply intertwined with the unrelenting pursuit of physical perfection. This exploration reveals the roots of their popularity among athletes and the insider secrets behind their remarkable ability to sculpt imposing physiques and catapult athletic performance.

However, before we dive deeper into the enigma of these synthetic marvels, it is imperative that we unravel the intricate orchestration that unfolds within our biological domains. Steroids, masterful mimics of our endogenous hormonal cascade, choreograph a complex dance with our endocrine system. Within the domain of anabolic steroids, we find a realm of hypertrophic growth, where muscle hypertrophy and bone density are sculpted with a nearly divine precision. Our journey takes us to the very core of this scientific enterprise, dissecting the mechanisms governing the actions of steroids and unveiling the blessings and curses they bestow upon those who venture down their path.

Within this complex mixture of human biology and chemical ingenuity, we must distinguish between two profoundly divergent classes of steroids: anabolic steroids, the champions of hypertrophy and physique enhancement, and corticosteroids, the couriers of therapeutic relief within the medical arena. Each class serves a unique purpose, demanding a meticulous examination that extends beyond the boundaries of bodybuilding.

However, as our voyage continues, we find ourselves at the crossroads of ethics, legality, and health. The choices laid before us are as personal as they are pivotal, and the looming question of legality casts a formidable shadow, leaving individuals to navigate a labyrinthine world of regulations and restrictions that vary across national borders. The choices we make are fraught with consequences both overt and latent.

But, dear reader, our journey does not culminate with the mere exposition of science or the condemnation of ethics. It culminates in a call for informed deliberation, for the synthesis of knowledge, ethics, and aspiration. The path toward achieving fitness and performance aspirations is multifaceted, and the allure of steroids is but one facet, glistening with both promise and peril.

The secrets of steroids may be unveiled, but the true revelation lies in the choices we make, the consequences we accept, and the stance we ultimately adopt in our unwavering pursuit of personal and athletic excellence. Let us embark on this voyage not as passive observers but as discerning travelers on the road to enlightenment, empowered by knowledge and guided by an unwavering compass of ethics and wisdom, fueled by research that forms the bedrock of our understanding. Shrouded in mystery, clouded by myths, are steroids actually effective for strength training? Or are they just a hoax that fuels a million dollar industry? And if they are so potent, do they actually have those side effects that many claim? This and much more will come to your knowledge in the following chapter!

***

Steroids and Their Role in Bodybuilding

In the world of bodybuilding, the discussion of steroids is both ubiquitous and polarizing. These synthetic compounds, which replicate the effects of natural hormones, particularly testosterone, have been a topic of intrigue and controversy for decades. Understanding their role in bodybuilding requires a nuanced exploration of the benefits, risks, and ethical considerations associated with their use.

The Anabolic Advantage:

The allure of steroids in bodybuilding lies in their anabolic properties. Anabolic steroids are aptly named, as they promote anabolism, the process of building and repairing muscle tissue. Here are some key ways in which steroids impact bodybuilding:

• Enhanced Muscle Growth: Anabolic steroids accelerate muscle protein synthesis, leading to faster and more substantial muscle gains. Bodybuilders can achieve a more muscular and defined physique in a shorter period.

• Increased Strength: Steroids enhance the body's ability to create new muscle fibers, resulting in increased strength. This strength boost is vital for lifting heavier weights and pushing the boundaries of one's training.

• Enhanced Recovery: Steroids can reduce muscle damage and inflammation, aiding in quicker recovery between workouts. This allows bodybuilders to train more frequently and intensively.

• Improved Endurance: Some steroids can increase red blood cell production, enhancing oxygen-carrying capacity, and thus endurance during workouts.

The Risks and Side Effects:

While the performance-enhancing effects of steroids are enticing, it is essential to recognize the potential drawbacks and health risks. These include:

• Health Risks: Steroid misuse can lead to a range of health issues, including liver damage, cardiovascular problems, hormonal imbalances, and psychiatric effects such as mood swings and aggression.

• Dependency: Some individuals may become psychologically dependent on steroids, which can lead to a vicious cycle of use and withdrawal.

• Legality: The use of steroids without a prescription is illegal in many countries, and athletes caught using them in competitions may face disqualification.

• Ethical Concerns: Steroid use can compromise

the fairness and integrity of competitive sports, as it provides an unfair advantage to those who use them.

Finding Your Stance:

The decision to use steroids in bodybuilding is highly personal and should be made after careful consideration of the potential benefits and risks. It is crucial to adopt a well-informed and ethical approach to this choice:

• Education: Before considering steroid use, individuals should educate themselves about the different types of steroids, potential side effects, and safe usage guidelines.

• Consultation: Seeking guidance from medical professionals and experienced trainers can provide valuable insights into the potential risks and benefits.

• Legal and Ethical Considerations: Understand the legal and ethical implications of steroid use in your region and within the context of competitive sports.

• Alternatives: Explore alternative approaches to achieving your fitness goals, such as proper nutrition, training, and recovery strategies, as these can yield significant results without the risks associated with steroids.

To sum it up, steroids have a well-established role in bodybuilding, offering the potential for enhanced muscle growth and performance. However, their use is not without risks and ethical considerations. Making an informed decision, guided by knowledge and a commitment to health and integrity, is essential for anyone contemplating the use of steroids in the pursuit of their bodybuilding goals.

***

Understanding How Steroids Interact with Your Biology

In the realm of bodybuilding and sports performance enhancement, a crucial aspect is comprehending how steroids interact with your biology. Anabolic steroids, in particular, are designed to mimic the effects of the male sex hormone testosterone. These synthetic compounds wield a powerful influence on the body's hormonal system, impacting various physiological processes. Here, we delve into the intricacies of how steroids interact with your biology.

- **The Hormonal Orchestra:**

At the heart of understanding steroids' effects is grasping their orchestration of the hormonal symphony within your body. Anabolic steroids, as the name suggests, promote anabolism, which is the process of building and repairing tissues. The key aspects of this interaction include:

- Testosterone Imitation: Anabolic steroids closely resemble the structure of testosterone, binding to androgen receptors in the cells. This binding activates a cascade of reactions, ultimately leading to the synthesis of proteins and the growth of muscle tissue.

• Muscle Protein Synthesis: One of the primary mechanisms is an increase in the rate of muscle protein synthesis. This means that the body creates muscle proteins at a faster rate, resulting in muscle growth and recovery.

• Bone Density and Erythropoiesis: Steroids also promote the growth and maintenance of bone density, and some can stimulate the production of red blood cells, improving oxygen transport to muscles. These effects enhance endurance and overall performance.

• **The Anabolic vs. Androgenic Effects:**
It's important to distinguish between the anabolic and androgenic effects of steroids. Anabolic effects are related to muscle growth and repair, while androgenic effects pertain to the development of male sexual characteristics. The ratio of anabolic to androgenic effects varies among different steroids.

• Anabolic Effects: These are responsible for the muscle-building and performance-enhancing properties of steroids. They increase muscle mass, strength, and endurance.

• Androgenic Effects: These effects can lead to the development of male traits, such as a deepening voice, facial hair growth, and changes in libido. Excessive androgenic effects can lead to virilization in women.

• **Hormone Regulation:**

The endocrine system, which regulates hormones in the body, plays a pivotal role in this interaction. The use of anabolic steroids can disrupt the natural balance of hormones, particularly the production of endogenous testosterone. This disruption can lead to a range of potential side effects, including testicular atrophy and infertility.

- **Individual Variability:**

It's crucial to recognize that the interaction between steroids and one's biology can vary significantly from person to person. Genetic factors, age, and overall health can all influence how the body responds to steroid use. Some individuals may experience more significant gains in muscle mass and strength, while others may be more prone to side effects.

In summary, understanding how steroids interact with your biology is essential for anyone considering their use. While these compounds can yield significant benefits in terms of muscle growth and athletic performance, their effects on the endocrine system and the potential for side effects must not be underestimated. Making an informed decision about steroid use involves a thorough comprehension of these interactions, coupled with a commitment to responsible and safe usage, if one chooses to go down that path.

***

The Choices, the Consequences, and Finding Your Stance

When pursuing bodybuilding, individuals often confront a significant crossroads in their journey towards achieving their fitness goals: the decision to use steroids. This decision is deeply personal and carries far-reaching consequences that extend beyond the confines of the gym. The process of finding your stance on this matter necessitates a judicious consideration of ethical, legal, and health-related factors.

- **The Choices:**

The decision to incorporate steroids into one's bodybuilding regimen is one of profound significance. It has the potential to significantly impact one's pursuit of the desired physique and athletic performance. This process of choice involves several key considerations:

- Fitness Objectives: It is paramount to assess one's fitness objectives. Whether the goal is to compete at a professional level or enhance personal physique, these goals will fundamentally influence the approach to steroid use.

- Educational Foundation: Prior to making a decision, it is incumbent upon individuals to acquire a comprehensive understanding of the various types of steroids, their potential side effects, and the responsible guidelines governing their usage. An informed decision hinges on a solid knowledge base.

• Consultation: Seeking counsel from medical professionals and experienced trainers is invaluable. They can provide an expert assessment of whether steroid use aligns with one's fitness goals and overall health status.

• Legal Considerations: It is essential to investigate the legal status of steroids in one's jurisdiction. The use of steroids without a valid prescription is illegal in many regions, and transgressions may entail severe legal repercussions.

• **The Consequences:**

Every choice, including the decision to use steroids, carries a set of repercussions. These consequences span a spectrum of physical, legal, and ethical dimensions:

• Health Implications: Misuse of steroids can engender a gamut of health-related issues, including liver damage, cardiovascular complications, hormonal imbalances, and psychological effects like mood swings and aggression. A comprehensive comprehension of these health risks is of paramount importance.

• Legal Ramifications: The utilization of steroids without a prescription is prohibited in numerous jurisdictions. Individuals found in possession may encounter legal penalties, including fines and potential incarceration.

• Dependency: A subset of users may develop a

psychological dependency on steroids, leading to a cycle of consumption and withdrawal. This can exert a profound impact on one's mental and emotional well-being.

• Ethical Dilemmas: Steroid use can introduce ethical quandaries, particularly concerning the fairness and integrity of competitive sports. This moral quandary extends to issues of fairness and respect within the bodybuilding community.

• **Finding Your Stance:**

As one navigates the complex terrain of choices and their accompanying consequences, the process of finding a personal stance on the use of steroids in bodybuilding is paramount. Several guiding principles should be considered:

• Informed Decision-Making: Base your choices on a foundation of knowledge and comprehension. Carefully weigh the potential advantages and disadvantages.

• Legal and Ethical Considerations: Understand and adhere to the legal and ethical consequences of steroid use within your geographical region and within the context of competitive sports.

• Exploration of Alternatives: Embrace and explore alternative avenues to realize your fitness objectives, such as prudent nutrition, rigorous training, and effective recovery strategies. These methods can yield significant results without the attendant risks associated with steroids.

• Alignment with Personal Values: Ultimately, your stance should align with your personal values and principles. Contemplate your ethical framework and the ramifications of your choices on both your individual life and the broader fitness community.

In summary, the process of navigating the choices, consequences, and finding your stance on steroid use in bodybuilding is intricately entwined with your pursuit of fitness goals. The process of making an informed and ethical choice necessitates a careful evaluation of potential benefits and risks, an appreciation of legal implications, and the acceptance of alternative pathways to achieving your objectives. Your stance should mirror your values and priorities as you traverse the multifaceted landscape of bodybuilding and performance enhancement.

"Don't let a person pressure you into taking steroids and don't let a person pressure you out of it. It's your life not theirs!"

6 DEBUNKING MYTHS AND EMBRACING TRUTHS

In the bodybuilding world, myths and truths are like the twin titans that govern the destiny of every aspiring sculptor of muscle. With biceps as big as boulders and chests that could rival the mountains, bodybuilders have long been the embodiment of raw power and physical perfection. Yet, beneath the gleaming sheen of sweat and the clanking of iron, a cacophony of misconceptions and half-truths has echoed through the ages. With this chapter, we move deeper into the heart of this iron jungle, armed not with fables and fantasies but with the sharpest sword of knowledge, ready to cut through the vines of falsehood that entwine the minds of many.

It's time to strip away the layers of illusion, revealing the naked truth that is the essence of bodybuilding — the science, the sweat, and the spirit behind each rep and each drop of perspiration. Welcome to the realm of "Debunking Myths and Embracing Truths," where the iron never lies, and the journey to greatness begins with the power of understanding.

***

Since I set my eyes on perfecting my body, I obviously met a lot of people from the same field; a couple of them had spent a few years already in the bodybuilding scenario, and others were still fresh; one thing I realized as I conversed with them was — myths and misconception attached to bodybuilding. Though I didn't believe them, as an amateur, you, at times, get inspired and impacted. To save you and other aspirants from going down the wrong track. Let's begin with the part where we debunk the myths that have either been created recently or over the decades.

Myth 1: "Lifting Heavy Weights Makes You Bulky"

Debunked: One of the most persistent myths in bodybuilding is the belief that lifting heavy weights will automatically turn you into a hulking behemoth. In reality, this is far from the truth. Building substantial muscle mass, or hypertrophy, involves genetics, nutrition, and training intensity. Lifting heavy weights is just one piece of the puzzle.

To debunk this myth, consider that muscular hypertrophy primarily depends on your diet and training program. Heavy lifting can contribute to muscle growth, but it will only cause you to become bulky if you intentionally consume a significant surplus of calories. The key to achieving a lean and toned physique is to focus on a well-balanced diet and training program incorporating heavy resistance training and higher-repetition, lower-weight exercises. This approach will help sculpt your muscles without bulking you up unnecessarily.

Myth 2: "Spot Reduction Burns Fat in Target Areas"

Debunked: Many people believe that performing exercises that target specific areas of the body, such as crunches for the abdomen or leg lifts for the thighs, will miraculously burn fat in those particular areas. Unfortunately, spot reduction is a myth. Your body doesn't selectively burn fat from the region you're working out.

In reality, fat loss occurs systemically and is influenced by factors like genetics and overall calorie expenditure. By creating a calorie deficit through diet and exercise, your body will gradually shed fat from various areas. It's essential to focus on a balanced approach that includes cardiovascular exercise, strength training, and a healthy diet to achieve overall fat loss and reveal the muscles beneath.

Myth 3: "More Protein Equals More Muscle"

Debunked: While protein is a crucial component of muscle growth and repair, the idea that consuming excessive amounts of protein will lead to larger muscles needs to be clarified. Your body is limited to how much protein it can utilize for muscle building.

Protein requirements vary from person to person and depend on age, gender, activity level, and goals. Consuming more protein than your body can use does not lead to bigger muscles. In fact, excessive protein intake can be stored as fat or lead to other health issues. To optimize muscle growth, focus on consuming an adequate amount of protein that aligns with your individual needs and engage in consistent resistance training.

Myth 4: "Carbohydrates Are the Enemy of Muscle Building"

Debunked: Carbohydrates often get a bad rap when it comes to bodybuilding, with some believing that they should be avoided to achieve a lean, muscular physique. This is a myth. Carbohydrates are a primary source of energy, especially during intense workouts.

Carbs provide the fuel your muscles need to perform optimally, and they play a crucial role in post-workout recovery. Restricting carbs too severely can lead to fatigue, hinder muscle growth, and reduce workout performance. Instead, focus on consuming the right balance of carbohydrates to support your energy and recovery needs while working towards your bodybuilding goals.

Myth 5: "You Can Out-Train a Poor Diet"

Debunked: This myth is a common pitfall for many individuals pursuing bodybuilding. Some believe that intense workouts can compensate for an unhealthy diet, but the reality is that nutrition is paramount. You can't out-train a poor diet.

Your body's ability to build and maintain muscle, as well as lose fat, is heavily influenced by what you eat. To achieve your bodybuilding goals, it's essential to maintain a balanced and nutrient-rich diet that supports your training regimen. Proper nutrition fuels your workouts and aids in muscle recovery, making it an indispensable component of any successful bodybuilding journey.

Myth 6: "Muscle Turns Into Fat When You Stop Working Out"

Debunked: This is a common misconception, but it's entirely false. Muscle and fat are two distinct tissues with different functions. When you stop working out, your muscles may atrophy or decrease in size due to reduced stimulus, but they don't magically transform into fat. What often happens is that people who stop exercising may gain fat because they are burning fewer calories and not replacing the energy expenditure with muscle-building activities.

Myth 7: "Supplements Are a Shortcut to Success"

Debunked: While supplements can be beneficial in certain circumstances, they are not a magical shortcut to achieving your bodybuilding goals. There is no substitute for a balanced diet and a well-structured training program. Supplements should complement your diet and training, not replace them. Overreliance on supplements can be costly and may yield the desired results with a solid foundation of nutrition and exercise.

Myth 8: "Women Who Lift Weights Will Get Bulky"

Debunked: This myth often deters women from lifting weights out of fear of developing a bulky appearance. In reality, women typically lack the levels of testosterone required to bulk up like men. Strength training is incredibly beneficial for women and helps build lean muscle, increase metabolism, and improve body composition. It can lead to a toned and fit appearance, not excessive bulkiness.

Myth 9: "You Can 'Tone' Your Muscles"

Debunked: The concept of "toning" is often misunderstood. What people typically mean by toning is reducing body fat to reveal well-defined muscles. There's no separate exercise for "toning" muscles; it's about building lean muscle through resistance training and simultaneously losing body fat through a calorie deficit. Therefore, you can only tone muscles if you address your overall body composition.

Myth 10: "More Training Equals Faster Results"

Debunked: Overtraining can be counterproductive and even detrimental to your progress. Rest and recovery are essential for muscle growth and injury prevention. Training intensely every day without adequate recovery time can lead to burnout, increased risk of injury, and hindered progress. A well-structured training plan that includes rest days and proper recovery periods is crucial for long-term success in bodybuilding.

Myth 11: "Stretching Before Exercise Prevents Injuries"

Debunked: While stretching is valuable for improving flexibility and range of motion, static stretching before a workout may not prevent injuries and can even reduce muscle strength temporarily. Instead, it's more effective to perform dynamic warm-up exercises and save static stretching after your workout when muscles are warm and pliable.

***

Alright, folks, in our earlier discussions in this book, we've covered quite a bit about bodybuilding. We've delved into the science of muscle growth, the significance of nutrition, and the importance of well-structured training programs. But now, it's time to address a topic that's been buzzing in the bodybuilding community: the use of steroids, the side effects they can bring, and the safety concerns that come with them.

So, let's talk about steroids. They're synthetic derivatives of testosterone and are sometimes used in bodybuilding to get those fast and substantial gains. There's no denying that they can make you big and strong in a hurry. However, it's essential to be upfront about the ethical, legal, and health-related issues that come with them.

Now, when it comes to side effects, they can be a mixed bag, and it depends on various factors like the type and amount of steroids used, how long they're used, and how your body reacts. Some common side effects include things like acne, oily skin, hair loss (especially if you're genetically predisposed), and even the growth of breast tissue in men – which is often referred to as gynecomastia.

But it's not just physical; there are psychological side effects, too. Mood swings, aggression, and irritability can rear their heads, and in some cases, steroids have been linked to severe psychiatric symptoms.

On the health front, steroids can mess with your cardiovascular system, affecting your cholesterol levels and raising your blood pressure. They might also strain your liver, mainly if you're using oral steroids, which can lead to liver damage or disease.

Hormonal imbalances are another concern. Steroids can throw your natural hormone balance out of whack, potentially affecting testosterone production and, in some instances, causing infertility.

Then there's the matter of dependency and withdrawal. Prolonged steroid use can lead to both physical and psychological dependence, and when you stop, withdrawal symptoms can be a real challenge.

And let's not forget the legal and ethical consequences. Using steroids without a prescription is illegal in many countries, and that could land you in legal trouble, facing fines or even imprisonment. In the realm of sports, using steroids can lead to disqualification and damage an athlete's reputation. It raises ethical concerns, too, especially about fair competition.

In terms of safety, there's a lot at stake. The health risks related to steroid use are significant and can have long-lasting consequences. The legality factor can't be ignored either; using or possessing steroids without a prescription is against the law in many places. Ethical concerns are also on the table, particularly the message it sends to young and impressionable individuals.

So, the bottom line is this: the potential risks that come with steroids far outweigh any short-term gains they may promise. We've discussed the importance of dedication to proper nutrition, structured training programs, rest, and patience in your bodybuilding journey. These are your best and safest bet for success.

If you're an aspiring bodybuilder, seeking guidance from qualified trainers and nutritionists, setting realistic expectations, and taking a holistic approach that prioritizes your health and well-being is the way to go. While steroids might seem tempting to some, remember that real and lasting progress is best achieved by committing to your long-term health and integrity.

Steroids, specifically anabolic-androgenic steroids (AAS), can indeed affect the male reproductive system, but their effects on penis and testicular size are often misunderstood. The primary role of the testes is to produce testosterone and sperm. When external testosterone (from AAS use) is introduced, the body's natural production of testosterone can decrease because the testes no longer need to produce as much, if any, testosterone. As a result, the testicles might temporarily decrease in size. This phenomenon is not due to a decrease in testosterone but rather a decrease in the need for the testes to actively produce it. Much like the body's response to cold temperatures, where the testes retract closer to the body for optimal sperm and testosterone production, the decrease in testicular size can be observed.

Contrary to common belief, there is no scientific evidence suggesting that steroid use directly reduces penis size. In fact, prolonged use of testosterone can potentially lead to an increase in penile size due to increased blood flow and tissue growth, though these effects can vary among individuals. Additionally, the enlargement of the clitoris in female bodybuilders who use testosterone or other androgenic substances is an example of androgenic effects on external genitalia. This occurs because the clitoris contains erectile tissue similar to the penis, and increased androgen levels can stimulate growth in this tissue. It's crucial to note that the use of steroids, especially without medical supervision, can lead to a myriad of adverse health effects beyond changes in reproductive organs. These can include cardiovascular issues, hormonal imbalances, liver damage, psychiatric effects, and more.

Seeking professional guidance from healthcare providers or endocrinologists is essential before considering or using any form of steroids. Understanding the potential risks and effects on the body's hormonal balance is crucial for informed decision-making regarding steroid use.

It's hard to see overweight people in the gym doing abs or trying to spot reduce fat. Just remember that you read this book and you are ahead of the game.

7 AMPLIFYING GAINS: LEGAL SUPPLEMENTS FOR THE WIN

Alright, folks, buckle up and get comfy because we're about to deep-dive into the world of legal supplements. This isn't your run-of-the-mill supplements 101; we're talking about the real deal— the ones that won't get you flagged on a doping test or raise eyebrows at the gym.

Let's start with the nitty-gritty: what makes a supplement "legal"? Well, legality here means these products have ingredients that are permitted by sports organizations, health authorities, and the law itself. They're the good guys of the supplement world, no questionable substances hiding in the shadows.

Now, here's a jaw-dropping stat to set the stage: the global supplement industry is soaring to unprecedented heights, reaching a staggering $200 billion by 2026! That's more dough than the GDP of some small countries. And guess what? Legal supplements are a major driving force in this cosmic growth spurt, proving that you can achieve gains galore without any legal headaches.

But let's not get lost in the numbers game. This journey is all about finding your fitness sidekick—the Robin to your Batman. From protein powders that'll turn you into a muscle-building machine to pre-workouts that'll rev your engines before hitting the treadmill, legal supplements cover a vast landscape of fitness support.

Think of legal supplements as your reliable gym buddies—always there to give you that extra edge without the risk of getting sidelined. They're the secret weapons in your arsenal, designed to boost performance, aid recovery, and keep you on the right side of the law and fitness goals.

So, grab a seat and get ready for an eye-opening exploration. We're dissecting, demystifying, and uncovering the universe of legal supplements so you can make informed choices and conquer your fitness odyssey without any shady shortcuts. Get ready to flex those muscles—the legal way!

Identifying legal supplements amidst the sea of options can feel like navigating a maze, but fear not, there are ways to distinguish the good from the questionable. Firstly, legality often boils down to the ingredients. Legal supplements contain components approved by regulatory bodies like the FDA, ensuring they comply with established safety and efficacy standards. You'll often find them in reputable stores, endorsed by recognizable brands, and displaying transparent labels listing their ingredients.

Now, about those illegal supplements lurking in the fitness realm—oh yes, they exist. These renegades often contain banned substances or undisclosed ingredients that could get you in hot water with sports authorities or pose health risks. Sometimes marketed as "miracle" solutions promising superhuman results, they're the rebels of the supplement world, promising the moon but delivering trouble instead.

The perks of sticking to legal supplements are manifold. Firstly, peace of mind—no need to worry about failed drug tests or unexpected health issues. They're designed to enhance your performance within safe limits, offering support without risking your well-being or reputation. Plus, legality ensures accountability. Companies producing legal supplements are held to strict standards, fostering transparency in their manufacturing processes and ingredient sourcing.

Moreover, legal supplements are often backed by

research and science, meaning you're investing in products with proven effectiveness. They're the reliable workhorses of the fitness world, aiding in muscle recovery, boosting energy levels, and supporting overall fitness goals without veering into dicey territories.

So, think of legal supplements as your trusty sidekick, standing by your fitness journey without the drama. They're the smart choice for those seeking gains without the headaches—keeping you on the right track towards your fitness zenith!

****

When it comes to maximizing fat loss and muscle gains, science-backed aids can be game-changers in your fitness arsenal. Let's delve into these supportive aids that have research-backed evidence supporting their efficacy. However, one thing like always, remember, while these aids have scientific backing, they work best when complemented with a balanced diet and consistent exercise routine. Additionally, it's essential to consult with a healthcare professional or a certified nutritionist before starting any supplement regimen to ensure they align with your health goals and overall well-being.

Picture this: you're on a fitness quest, and legal supplements are your trusted companions, each playing a unique role in sculpting your dream physique. As you embark on this journey, armed with science-backed aids, you're about to unlock a realm of potential where gains and losses transform into your fitness masterpiece.

- **Protein Supplements:**

Goals: Protein supplements aim to support muscle recovery, aid in muscle growth, and fulfill daily protein requirements, especially for individuals with higher protein needs due to intense workouts or limited dietary sources.

Benefits: They provide a convenient way to increase protein intake, aiding in muscle repair after workouts, enhancing muscle protein synthesis, reducing muscle soreness, and supporting overall muscle growth and maintenance.

- **Creatine:**

Goals: Creatine is geared towards increasing muscle strength, improving exercise performance, and supporting high-intensity workouts.

Benefits: Its supplementation increases phosphocreatine stores in muscles, promoting ATP production, leading to improved muscle strength and power, enhanced muscle mass, increased workout capacity, and quicker recovery between sets.

- **Caffeine:**

Goals: Caffeine is used to boost energy levels, increase focus and alertness during workouts, and promote fat burning.

Benefits: It stimulates the central nervous system, increasing metabolism, improving mental focus and endurance, reducing perceived exertion during exercise, and enhancing fat oxidation, potentially aiding in weight loss.

- **Branched-Chain Amino Acids (BCAAs):**

Goals: BCAAs aim to stimulate muscle protein synthesis, reduce muscle soreness, and prevent muscle breakdown during intense exercise.

Benefits: They assist in reducing muscle breakdown, enhancing muscle recovery, reducing fatigue during workouts, preserving lean muscle mass, and supporting overall muscle growth.

- **Beta-Alanine:**

Goals: Beta-Alanine aims to increase muscle carnosine levels, thereby delaying muscle fatigue and improving endurance during high-intensity exercise.

Benefits: Its supplementation results in improved muscle endurance, reduced fatigue during repetitive high-intensity exercises, increased training volume, and enhanced performance in activities lasting 1-4 minutes.

- **Fish Oil (Omega-3 Fatty Acids):**

Goals: Omega-3 fatty acids from fish oil support joint health, reduce muscle soreness, and aid in muscle recovery.

Benefits: They possess anti-inflammatory properties, promoting joint flexibility, reducing exercise-induced inflammation and muscle soreness, supporting cardiovascular health, and potentially enhancing muscle recovery.

- **Vitamin D:**

Goals: Vitamin D aims to support muscle function, aid in recovery, and promote overall health.

Benefits: Its supplementation helps improve muscle strength, reduce the risk of injury, support immune function, and potentially aid in weight management and fat loss.

***

Nurturing your body naturally through a mindful approach to health often involves a comprehensive and holistic strategy encompassing various practices, including maintaining a balanced diet, engaging in regular exercise, ensuring adequate sleep, managing stress levels, and sometimes incorporating supplements to support overall well-being. The journey to optimal health is multifaceted, and the role of supplements is just one piece of the puzzle.

Here's a more detailed exploration of how you can nurture your body naturally, one supplement at a time:

- Holistic Health Approach: Adopting a holistic approach means considering the interconnectedness of various aspects of health. It's about understanding that good nutrition, physical activity, mental wellness, adequate rest, and healthy lifestyle choices collectively contribute to overall well-being.

- Importance of Nutritious Diet: The foundation of a healthy lifestyle is a well-balanced and diverse diet. Consuming a variety of nutrient-dense foods such as fruits, vegetables, whole grains, lean proteins, and healthy fats provides essential vitamins, minerals, antioxidants, and other vital nutrients necessary for optimal body function.

• Supplements as Support: While obtaining nutrients from food is ideal, sometimes dietary restrictions, certain health conditions, or lifestyle choices might lead to nutrient deficiencies. Supplements can act as a complement to fill these gaps. For example, vitamin D for those with limited sun exposure or omega-3 fatty acids for individuals not consuming enough fatty fish.

• Consulting Healthcare Professionals: Before starting any supplement regimen, seeking guidance from healthcare professionals, such as doctors, registered dietitians, or nutritionists, is crucial. They can provide personalized advice based on individual health needs, ensuring that supplements are safe, effective, and appropriate.

• Quality and Safety: Opting for supplements from reputable brands that undergo rigorous quality testing and adhere to safety standards is paramount. Third-party certifications, like USP, NSF, or ConsumerLab, can indicate quality and purity.

• Understanding Dosage and Interactions: It's essential to follow recommended dosages and be aware of potential interactions between supplements and medications. Some supplements may interfere with prescription drugs or have adverse effects if taken in excess.

• Patience and Consistency: Supplements may take time to show their effects. Consistency in taking them as directed is crucial for experiencing potential benefits. Regular monitoring and adjustments, if necessary, are also vital aspects of a supplement regimen.

• Individual Variations: Each person's body is unique. Factors like genetics, age, gender, health conditions, and lifestyle choices influence how supplements may work for an individual.

• Periodic Check-ups: Regular evaluations with healthcare providers can help monitor progress, reassess needs, and adjust supplement regimens accordingly. These check-ups ensure that the supplements continue to support overall health effectively.

In summary, nurturing your body naturally involves a comprehensive approach that includes a balanced diet, regular exercise, adequate rest, stress management, and occasionally, supplements when necessary. Always prioritize a healthy lifestyle as the foundation for well-being, with supplements acting as supportive elements to help maintain optimal health.

8 THE JOURNEY'S END AND NEW BEGINNINGS

This book delves deeply into the science behind muscle development, offering a comprehensive understanding of how muscles grow and the factors influencing this process. It breaks down complex concepts into simpler terms, explaining the chemical mechanisms at play and providing valuable insights into optimizing muscle growth potential. The emphasis is on empowering readers with knowledge to make informed choices about their fitness journey.

Beyond muscle growth, the book places a significant focus on weight loss and boosting self-confidence. It isn't just about shedding pounds but also about fostering a positive self-image. It explores various avenues for weight loss, including supplements, dietary strategies, and even touches upon the controversial topic of steroids. However, the underlying message resonates with the importance of inner transformation, advocating for feeling good internally along with external changes.

Workouts take a central role, exploring different types and their specific benefits. Whether it's powerlifting, CrossFit, or other exercise regimens, the book provides insights into choosing a workout routine that suits individual preferences and goals. Importantly, it emphasizes setting realistic goals and acknowledging progress, regardless of its scale, as a vital component of the journey.

Dietary diversity is another key area covered extensively. It scrutinizes various diets such as keto, fasting, and low glycemic diets, discussing their impacts on the body and how they contribute to muscle building and overall health. By weighing the pros and cons of different dietary approaches, the book equips readers with the knowledge to make informed choices about their nutrition.

Steroids, a topic often surrounded by controversy, are addressed candidly. The book educates readers on how steroids work, their potential effects, and the risks involved. It aims to provide clarity and understanding so individuals can make educated decisions regarding their use.

Furthermore, the book addresses prevalent myths

and misconceptions in the realm of bodybuilding. It seeks to debunk misconceptions, particularly about safety concerns and the realities of achieving certain body goals. The emphasis lies on honesty and authenticity throughout the fitness journey.

Lastly, legal supplements are discussed as aids in achieving fitness goals. The book explores the world of scientifically-backed supplements that can assist in muscle growth and fat loss, advocating for natural methods to support the body's progress.

In summary, this book offers a comprehensive and holistic approach to fitness, encompassing scientific knowledge, personalized strategies, and ethical considerations. It encourages individuals to understand their bodies, work hard towards their goals, and maintain a balanced approach that nurtures both physical health and mental well-being. The overarching message revolves around embarking on a fitness journey that is realistic, sustainable, and prioritizes overall health.

***

As we draw towards the end of this book, Understanding nutrition, bodybuilding, and the role of steroids in the context of fitness and health provides a holistic view that considers various aspects of physical development and well-being.

Nutrition: Nutrition forms the foundation of any fitness journey. It's not just about counting calories but rather understanding the role of different nutrients in fueling the body. A balanced diet comprising proteins, carbohydrates, fats, vitamins, and minerals is essential for overall health and energy. In the context of bodybuilding, nutrition becomes even more crucial as it directly influences muscle growth, repair, and recovery. The right balance and timing of nutrients can significantly impact performance during workouts and the body's ability to develop and maintain muscle mass.

Bodybuilding: Bodybuilding is not solely about sculpting a physique but involves discipline, consistency, and dedication towards achieving fitness goals. It encompasses various aspects such as tailored workout routines, proper nutrition, adequate rest, and mental focus. It's about setting realistic goals, working hard, and celebrating incremental progress. Building muscle requires a combination of resistance training, appropriate nutrition, and sufficient rest for muscles to recover and grow stronger. A holistic approach to bodybuilding involves understanding individual limitations, focusing on form and technique, and ensuring overall well-being alongside physical development.

Steroids: The use of steroids in bodybuilding is a controversial topic. Steroids, or performance-enhancing drugs, can have profound effects on muscle growth and recovery. However, they also come with potential risks and side effects that can impact overall health. Understanding the science behind steroids is crucial to make informed decisions. While some individuals may consider their use to expedite muscle growth, it's important to weigh the short-term gains against the potential long-term consequences. Building a well-informed perspective on steroids involves acknowledging their effects, risks, legality, and ethical considerations. It's about understanding that achieving fitness goals should not compromise overall health and well-being.

In essence, a holistic perspective on nutrition, bodybuilding, and the role of steroids in fitness revolves around balance, knowledge, and mindfulness. It's about nurturing the body through proper nutrition, embracing a disciplined approach to training, and making informed decisions regarding any external aids such as steroids, all while prioritizing long-term health and well-being over short-term gains. Achieving fitness goals should align with promoting overall health, emphasizing a balanced and sustainable approach to physical development.

***

Alright, before we finally conclude, let's talk about taking the reins and designing the body and fitness journey that's perfect for you. This idea is all about understanding that you're the architect of your bodybuilding and fitness expedition. It means having the power to make choices that lead to your desired physique. So, let's break it down.

When it comes to fitness, it's like having this incredible canvas in front of you, and you get to choose what you want to create. That could mean choosing workout routines that match your style and preferences – whether you're into lifting heavy or prefer more dynamic exercises like CrossFit. It's about finding what clicks for you.

Then there's the food part – the fuel for your body. You've got a palette full of choices: healthy proteins, good carbs, essential fats, and all the nutrients that support your fitness goals. It's understanding how these choices impact your body, giving you the energy and strength to push through your workouts and grow those muscles.

And guess what? Every decision counts. Every time you lace up your sneakers for a workout, choose a nutritious meal, or opt for rest to recover, you're taking a step toward your fitness goals. It's like putting a piece of the puzzle in place to create the bigger picture – your future self, strong, fit, and healthy.

This phrase is all about recognizing your power to create the body and fitness journey you want. It's about embracing the process, enjoying the journey, and celebrating every little victory along the way. Because in the end, it's your journey, your body, and your future you're crafting – and that's pretty amazing!

ABOUT THE AUTHOR

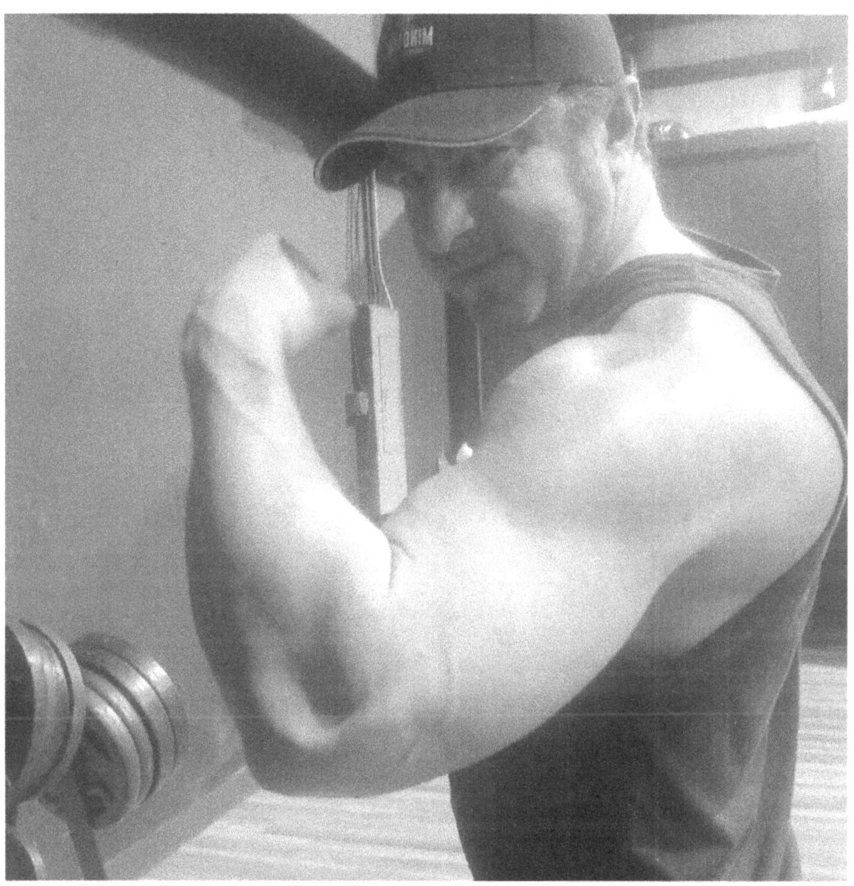

Jonathan Wright grew up in the small town of Wurtsboro NY. As a child he was obsessed with martial arts and fitness. With over 30 years of experience in martial arts and the fitness industry he is now deciding to share his experience and knowledge with the world.